DENTAL
EVIDENCE

DENTAL EVIDENCE

A HANDBOOK FOR POLICE

By

IRL A. GLADFELTER, D.D.S.

Member, American Society of Forensic Odontology
Member, International Society for Forensic Odonto-Stomatology
Chairman, Dental Section, Department of Surgery, Oak Park Hospital,
Oak Park, Illinois
Former Adjunct Attending, Section of Dental and Oral Surgery,
Department of Otolaryngology and Bronchoesophagology
Rush Presbyterian-St. Luke's Medical Center, Chicago, Illinois
Former Instructor, Department of Otolaryngology and Bronchoesophagology,
Rush Medical School, Chicago, Illinois

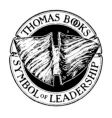

CHARLES C THOMAS • PUBLISHER
Springfield • Illinois • U.S.A.

Published and Distributed Throughout the World by

CHARLES C THOMAS · PUBLISHER

BANNERSTONE HOUSE

301-327 East Lawrence Avenue, Springfield, Illinois, U.S.A.

© *1975 by* CHARLES C THOMAS · PUBLISHER

ISBN 0-398-03323-4

Library of Congress Catalog Card Number: 74-17411

With THOMAS BOOKS *careful attention is given to all details of manufacturing and design. It is the Publisher's desire to present books that are satisfactory as to their physical qualities and artistic possibilities and appropriate for their particular use.* THOMAS BOOKS *will be true to those laws of quality that assure a good name and good will.*

Printed in the United States of America

Y-2

Library of Congress Cataloging in Publication Data

Gladfelter, Irl A.
  Dental evidence.

  Bibliography: p.
  1. Teeth—Identification. 2. Criminal investigation. 3. Evidence, Criminal. I. Title.
  [DNLM: 1. Forensic dentistry. W705 G542d]
  HV8073.5.G55   364.12′5   74-17411
  ISBN 0-398-03323-4

DEDICATION

*To my children, Irl Allen III and Mathew Ord,
and all children who are small now, in the hope that the
world we give them in twenty years will be safer
and more just through the efforts of our generation.*

FOREWORD

Forensic odontology, while long established in Europe, is finally becoming recognized in America as a full branch of the Forensic Sciences. Identification by the use of dental records is becoming almost routine in some parts of the country. Bite mark evidence has been accepted in American courts and the subject is finally being taught in some American dental schools.

The usefulness of any kind of evidence is dependent to a large extent on the skills of the police officer and the evidence technician in its recognition and preservation, which in turn is contingent on the training and experience given these officials. This is especially true in the case of dental evidence, due to its often transient and perishable nature and the ease with which it may be overlooked.

In the past, there has been little or no training available for police in this field. The excellent textbooks on Forensic Odontology have, in the past, been addressed to the medical or dental professions, for the most part, and have always assumed varying amounts of prior knowledge of medicine and dentistry without which they were difficult to really comprehend.

Dental Evidence: A Handbook for Police, is the first book of Forensic Odontology to address itself specifically to the Police. It gives a broad view of the entire subject, from its origin in 1066 A.D. to the present. It tells what dental evidence is, what it looks like, when and in what circumstances it may be found, and what to do with it until it is turned over to a dentist for evaluation. It gives all of the dental and scientific background necessary for a police officer to work with dental evidence, including briefings in such subjects as dental anatomy, growth and development, dental physiology, and dental materials. As it describes each situation in which dental evidence may be important, it tells in step-by-step manner what should be done to properly record and preserve this type of evidence and how to handle and correctly manipulate the dental materials used to preserve this evidence. This book delineates the roles of the police officer, the dentist, and the medical examiner and includes samples of forensic dental charts and a recommended equipment list.

As the materials used to preserve dental evidence require skill to manipulate, the latter portion of *Dental Evidence* details in step-by-step manner, both how to use them and how not to use them; and when to use or not to use each type of material. The author describes both the major characteristics of these materials and their more troublesome idiosyncrasies, and how to avoid the difficulties that they can cause. In most cases each step involved is accompanied by an illustration.

Dental Evidence: A Handbook for Police, is a useful and practical reference book for police departments and police academies and may be used in Police Science curricula at the college level, as well as by the individual police officer who wishes to broaden his knowledge. It may also be used both as a field handbook and as a training and laboratory manual. For those interested in further readings in this subject there is a bibliography of books and journal articles from the international literature (printed in English) pertaining to the police aspects of Forensic Odontology.

As Forensic Odontology becomes more and more important in the United States, this book is one that will be most interesting and practical for all law enforcement officers.

HARRY BEHRMANN
Chairman, Department of Police Science Administration
Triton College, River Grove, Illinois
Former Chief of Police, Broadview, Illinois
Retired Special Agent, U.S. Federal Bureau
of Investigation

ACKNOWLEDGMENTS

I WISH TO ACKNOWLEDGE the assistance of Joseph Rigo, C.D.T., of Des Plaines, Illinois, for the use of his dental laboratory and equipment in the preparation of many of the photographs in this volume.

I wish to especially acknowledge the assistance of my wife, Barbara Gladfelter, B.A., who, with the aid of facts I supplied, constructed this book.

IRL A. GLADFELTER, D.D.S.

CONTENTS

xi

DENTAL
EVIDENCE

Chapter 1 ____ ___ ___ ___ ___ ___ ___ ___ ___ ___

SCOPE OF THE FIELD

___ ___ ___ ___ ___ ___ ___ ___ ___ ___ ___ ___

DENTAL EVIDENCE, in the form of oral portions of human remains or bite imprints on objects or persons gathered by police, dentists or other personnel and used in the solution of legal problems, constitutes a branch of the forensic sciences known as forensic dentistry or forensic odontology. Although sometimes considered a relatively new science, it has actually been around for a long time. Four famous historical cases are illustrative.

Nine hundred years ago the Normans in England under William the Conqueror realized the value of bite marks as personal identification. As a formal seal on public documents, King William utilized a large piece of wax attached to the document, which he would then bite. He had a very unusual and abnormal tooth alignment and his bite mark was considered to provide sufficient identification for his royal documents.

In 1775 in what would soon become the United States, Paul Revere, who was active in many fields of endeavor including dentistry, made a silver wire dental bridge for General Joseph Warren of the Massachusetts Militia. This general was in partial command of the American troops at the Battle of Breed's Hill, during which he was killed. The enemy British recovered his body, took his expensive uniform and insignia braid, and buried him unclothed along with an unidentified person wearing a farmer's frock coat.

For awhile General Warren was listed as missing in action and possibly killed, but he was not definitely presumed lost until items of his uniform and insignia turned up elsewhere. Ten months later, in 1776, American authorities found a grave bearing two bodies, one in a farmer's frock and one unclothed. The unclothed body was wearing a very elaborate dental bridge, and it was Paul Revere's identification of the bridge he had made for General

Warren a year earlier which led to his identification.

In 1850, seventy-four years later, in Boston one of the more celebrated cases in the history of forensic dentistry occurred, the Webster-Parkman murder case. Dr. John Webster was a professor at the Harvard Medical School. He was stylish, led an extravagant lifestyle and spent money lavishly, having inherited a considerable amount. When all his money was gone, Webster obtained a number of loans from his friend, Dr. George Parkman, a wealthy and socially prominent medical doctor who owned a great deal of land in Boston and frequently loaned money to people. Because of their friendship, Dr. Parkman was more liberal in his loans to Dr. Webster than he would have been to others. On the occasion of the last loan from Dr. Parkman, Webster gave his valuable gem collection as collateral.

When Webster again ran into money problems, he felt he could not go back to Parkman for a further loan, so he approached Robert Shaw, Dr. Parkman's brother-in-law. Dr. Webster asked Shaw to loan him a considerable amount of money and offered his gem collection as collateral. Shaw was aware that this same gem collection had been used as collateral for a loan from Dr. Parkman, so Shaw went to his brother-in-law and told him of Webster's behavior. Parkman, enraged, ran back to Webster, accused him of fraud and demanded immediate repayment of all of his outstanding loans. Webster very politely replied that he would repay Parkman if he would only come to his office at the Medical School the next day. Dr. Parkman went and was never seen again.

Now, about the time Parkman made the loan, he had gone to Dr. Nathan Keep, a dentist, to have a set of porcelain dentures made. Parkman had to have these dentures made in a very short period of time because of his social obligations, and Dr. Keep found it necessary to literally work day and night for a time in order to have these dentures ready by the deadline Parkman had set. He made the deadline, but just barely.

One week after Parkman disappeared, a janitor at the Harvard Medical School found a dismembered headless body in the washroom in Webster's office. Later that same day a search by members of the Boston Police found a crushed skull bearing a porcelain denture in the furnace of the building in which Webster had his office. Webster was immediately arrested.

At the trial the dentist recognized the dentures he had made for Parkman because he remembered the long and painful hours it took to construct them. He also remembered the unique characteristics of Parkman's lower jaw and the unusual modifications necessary in the dentures to accommodate them. As proof that the porcelain dentures were in the head when the head was put in the furnace, Dr. Keep testified that porcelain dentures absorb saliva and the amount of heat produced in the furnace would have turned the saliva to steam and caused the porcelain dentures to explode if they had not been insulated inside the head at the time it was placed in the furnace. Also, Dr. Keep testified that the amount of heat in the furnace would have caused the denture spring to snap unless it was protected from the intense heat by the tissues of the head. Webster was convicted and later executed.

In 1930, a more bizarre case in which dental evidence figured prominently occurred in Australia. Arthur Upfield was the author of a number of murder mysteries and worked as a boundary rider on the rabbitproof fence in Western Australia. One night, sitting around the campfire, he conceived the idea of a novel in which there would be no corpse. He discussed with a "Snowy" Rowles different ways in which a murder could be accomplished and the corpse disposed of so completely that there would be no trace left. The method at which Upfield and Rowles arrived was to first shoot the victim, then burn the corpse to ashes, sift all of the ashes through a sieve and separate the metal and bones. The metal would be treated in acid, and that metal which was not eaten up with the acid would be so disfigured as to be unrecognizable. The bones would be ground to dust and deposited on the pile of ash. The final step would be to shoot two kangaroos, burn them in the fire and grind most of their bones into dust, leaving enough fragments for the coroner's officials to find in order to avert suspicion.

In 1930 three men disappeared: Louis Carron, a Mr. Lloyd and a Mr. Ryan. The three were last seen heading out along the rabbit-proof fence in Western Australia in Ryan's truck in the company of Snowy Rowles. Nothing more was seen of Carron, Lloyd or Ryan until the rabbit fence boundary riders found a series of fires with heaps of ashes to the side and a number of incinerated bones. The police and the coroner were notified and the coroner found that the bones in the ash were mostly those of kangaroos. However, he found small fragments of human bone, including fragments of one human skull, one entire human tooth with an unfilled cavity preparation in it, seventeen intact artificial teeth from a denture but with no denture base, two gold dental clasps, two shoe buttons, ten metal clothes rivets and one piece of melted lead.

Since Rowles had returned with the truck but without the other three men, suspicion centered on him, and he was immediately arrested. After his arrest he twice attempted to commit suicide in his cell, once by hanging and once by taking strychnine.

Dr. Arthur W. Sims, a dentist of Hamilton, New Zealand, was called in because he had treated Carron in New Zealand before Carron had gone to Australia. Dr. Sims recognized Carron in some photographs taken before his death and pointed him out as his former patient. When shown the intact human tooth with the filling preparation in it, Sims recognized the type of cavity preparation as one of his own. The fact that it was unfilled was attributed to the fact that the metal he used in fillings was a metal which would melt at the temperatures likely to be found in a fire, because it contained a high percentage of lead. He identified the gold clasps as some that he had made for Carron and recognized the artificial teeth as having come from his office. The dentists in New Zealand for the most part used artificial denture teeth held to the denture by pins. Dr. Sims used diatoric (pinless) teeth. He attributed the fact that no denture base was found with these teeth to the fact that his dentures were made of the type of vulcanite rubber which would burn in the temperatures of the fire leaving a fine ash.

This dental evidence and other supportive evidence led to the conviction of Rowles, who was hung. Lloyd and Ryan were never found. Their remains presumably were in the ashes of the other campfires along the rabbit fence.

These are just a few of the more famous cases in which dental evidence has figured prominently. The application of dental science to problems in criminal law has been utilized extensively in Europe, particularly Scandinavia and Britain, for over 100 years, in Japan since 1900, and is taught in their dental schools. The subject is so refined in Sweden that the testimony only of a dentist, not a physician, is accepted in court on any aspect of dental evidence.

The United States has recently begun to use dental evidence increasingly and to teach it in dental schools. In a number of recent cases the American courts have not only allowed the presentation of dental evidence, but dental evidence has been primarily responsible for the convictions obtained. In 1972 and 1973 the courts in the state of Connecticut ruled that the taking of impressions of the teeth and the mouth for purposes of comparison with bite marks does not constitute forcing an individual to give testimony against himself but instead is in the same category as fingerprinting. In Illinois in 1973 the courts, for the first time in history, granted a dentist a search warrant so that impressions and casts of the teeth of a suspect could be obtained for use as evidence in a homicide case.

In the field of dental forensics, three specific circumstances are commonly considered objects of inquiry: first, the identification of human remains through dental records and evaluation of dental remnants; second, the collection, preservation, evaluation and interpretation of bite mark evidence in criminal cases; and third, the use of dental evidence in dental malpractice cases. The latter case is not a matter for consideration by this author in this text or elsewhere, nor does it usually apply to police. The importance of the identification of human remains and of bite mark evidence and their pertinance to police work cause them to stand as a subject apart both for the dentist and for the police who play the primary role in noticing, collecting and preserving this evidence.

The one individual who will be present in all instances when dental evidence may be found, whether the evidence consists of human remains found in various places or after mass disasters, or whether the evidence consists of bite marks on the persons of the victims of homicide, sex crimes, other crimes of violence or of child abuse, is the police officer. While it is of value for the dentist to be educated in dental forensics, it is not he, but the police officer who is in the vital, first-line position to recognize and preserve dental evidence. No one is in a better position in this regard; therefore, the police officer should become cognizant of the fact that dental evidence does exist and is present in many types of cases. He should know what this dental evidence is likely to consist of, when to look for it, when it is likely to be present, and both the police officer and the police evidence technician should know how to handle this type of evidence and preserve it for evaluation by a dentist.

The police officer and the evidence technician should be prepared to assist the dentist by photographing the human remains, bite marks or other dental evidence, by taking impressions of the evidence in the appropriate impression material when indicated, by setting up and dismantling any equipment required by the dentist, by assisting the dentist in obtaining records or photographs made before death in doubtful identification cases, and should fulfill the role of the liaison officer between the dentist and other officials in other agencies. The police evidence technician in particular should be aware of when to call a dentist for consultation and when such a dental consultation is not necessary.

The purpose of this handbook is to acquaint the police officer and the evidence technician with the general field of dental evidence and specifically to advise them when to look for dental evidence, in what situations and in what crimes dental evidence is likely to be found, in which situation it is likely to be valuable, and when it is found how to record and preserve it properly so that it can be evaluated by a dentist. A second purpose of this handbook is to acquaint the police officer and the police evidence technician with the materials used in recording and preserving of dental evidence and to explain in considerable detail the techniques involved in the use of these materials. A brief chapter on dental anatomy and physiology has been included to provide some very basic knowledge of the human dental apparatus and how it works. Some basic understanding of this is essential for any appreciation and comprehension of the field of dental evidence. Some techniques used in forensic dentistry are also used in other branches of the forensic sciences and are dealt with in much more detail in standard books of evidence technology or photography. Therefore, the chapters or sections of chapters dealing with these items will be general and brief.

Dental evidence can be a very powerful tool both for prosecution and for defense in criminal cases as well as an important aid in the solution of a number of other problems. However, of necessity, it cannot be used unless the police officer or the evidence technician is aware of the scope, technology and limitations of the field. Since much dental evidence is of a transitory or perishable nature, the police officer and the evidence technician will determine by their knowledge and use of the proper methods of collection, recording and preservation of this evidence whether or not it will have any validity when it finally reaches a dentist for evaluation. The aim of this handbook is to provide that knowledge

Chapter 2 ___ __ __ __ __ __ __ __ __

BASIC DENTAL CONCEPTS
— — — — — — — — — — — —

THE INTELLIGENT POLICE OFFICER or police evidence technician, although persuaded of the value of preserving and utilizing dental evidence and convinced that it is worthwhile for him to add this to his repertoire of crime-solving techniques, may approach the subject rather timorously, feeling that such a broad subject as dental technology is beyond the scope of his time or background limitations to learn. It is the intent of this author to show the police officer or evidence technician that dental evidence technology is not difficult and can be learned in a reasonable amount of time available to the officer with a reasonable amount of effort, and that an extensive background is valuable but not absolutely necessary.

All the background in dental science absolutely necessary to the police officer or evidence technician is found in this chapter. Included is information about what teeth are, what they look like, when they erupt, variations among the races, how the jaws are formed and function, and how the teeth function as units in the biting apparatus. This information is a part of the general field of dental anatomy and physiology, a very broad and complex field which actually constitutes in itself a subdivision of dental science as well as a specialty within the science of anatomy and is only adequately discussed in a lengthy textbook limited to this subject. The general subject of dental anatomy and physiology itself does not actually directly pertain to any aspect of law enforcement, but the concepts will be of use to the officer and the evidence technician in helping him to better understand the field of dental evidence. If the reader wishes additional information in this area, he should refer to any of the textbooks in this field included in the bibliography.

While the scientific information about the human dentition and the jaw structure and function serves primarily as background for the police officer, it will be of interest to the evidence-oriented officer to know what the dentist can do with his knowledge of these subjects.

Knowledge of age and racial characteristics of human dentition is primarily useful in the field of dental identification of human remains. With his knowledge of human dentition, it is possble for the dentist, after careful examination of the stage and degree of tooth eruption, wear of the teeth, condition of the gums, calcium and mineral content of the teeth (by laboratory tests) and state of the root and bones (by X-rays), to determine the age of the subject within a range.

In the case of an individual under twelve, the approximate age may be determined to within about three months. In the case of an individual over twelve, it is possible for the dentist to pinpoint the age of the individual to within nine months of the actual age. These determinations are possible because of the fact that the teeth are yet in a mixed dentition state; some teeth are in, others out, some still in the bone, and some roots have dissolved. In the case of an individual over the age of twenty-one, the determination of the individual's age is more difficult by dental means alone, although it is possible within approximately three years. The amount of wear the teeth undergo varies considerably from individual to individual, depending on such factors as coarseness of diet, nervous habits like nail-biting, finger-biting, chewing toothpicks or other objects, or occupational habits such as holding nails or pins or other objects between the teeth which can cause unusual patterns of wear and attrition; to correlate these with age is difficult. It is possible to achieve some idea of the age of a person over the age of twenty-one by analyzing X-rays to determine the amount of bone resorption due to gum disease, and by means of chemical analysis to determine the calcium content of teeth, which increases with age. These are only approximations, however, and the determination of age of an individual over the age of twenty-one with all permanent teeth in place must always be done in close correlation with other data supplied by the medical pathologist.

With his knowledge of human dentition, by examining the teeth and the general facial and bone structure of skeletonized or badly decomposed remains, the dentist can also arrive at a determination of the probable race of the subject. The race of an individual cannot be determined entirely from traits present in teeth and facial bones since there are often more variations within racial groups than between them. However, there are general characteristics of the teeth and the skull which can provide some indication of the race of the subject. This "evidence of race" is primarily supportive and should not be relied on to the exclusion of other factors, but should be included with other factors provided by the medical pathologist in order to accurately determine the subject's probable race.

Knowledge of jaw structure and function is primarily useful in the field of criminal identification through bite mark evidence. With his knowledge of jaw structure and function, it is possible for the dentist to sometimes identify a bite pattern and correlate it with impressions and bite registrations obtained from a suspect and determine whether or not the suspect was able to have produced a bite mark in question. Impressions and cast replicas of the upper and lower teeth are made of the suspect and mounted on a machine called an articulator with the aid of wax imprints made by the suspect so that the casts of his teeth can be mounted on the articulator in the same relationship to each other as his own mouth. With this instrument, it is then possible, by using tracings of the movements of the jaws of an individual obtained with another instrument called a face bow, to reproduce all of the possible jaw movements of an individual, and to reproduce experimentally in wax all types of bite marks and registrations this suspect is capable of making on an object shaped similar to the object or portion of the body bitten. From this, the dentist is able to determine with a high degree of probability whether or not it was possible for the suspect to have left the bite mark in question.

HUMAN DENTITION
Adult Dentition

The normal adult dentition consists of thirty-two teeth. Of these thirty-two teeth, eight are incisors. There are broad, flat, sharp teeth in the front of the mouth, the purpose of which is to bite food. The upper ones are approximately twice the width of the lower ones.

There are four canines, or eye teeth, two on each side. These are heavy, triangular or cone-shaped teeth, with very long, slightly flattened roots. They are very important teeth and are sometimes called the "keystones" or "cornerstones" of the arch, and their function is to grip and tear food.

There are eight bicuspids or premolars, which are relatively small, trapezoidal teeth, with two elevations or cusps, one on the outside, or buccal, and one on the tongue side, or lingual. Their function is to grind food. These are small and relatively weak teeth and are occasionally congenitally missing or may be extracted for orthodontic purposes as they are not nearly as important as the other teeth in the mouth.

The remaining teeth are called molars. Molars are very large teeth with from three to five cusps on them, depending on their location in the arch and whether they are upper or lower teeth. Lower first molars generally have five cusps. The other lower molars generally have four. Upper molars generally have four cusps, but occasionally may have three. The function of the molar teeth is to grind food. They are heavy, massive teeth. Lower molars have two roots, and upper molars have three roots. An exception is found in individuals of Mongoloid race (Orientals, American Indians and Eskimos) who occasionally have lower molars with three roots.

The first permanent teeth to emerge into the oral cavity are the lower first molars. These are sometimes called six-year molars because of the age at which they appear. The upper first molars follow the eruption of the lowers by two to six months.

The second permanent teeth to come in are the lower central incisors. These are followed by the upper central incisors, and then the lower lateral incisors, then the upper lateral incisors.

The first premolars follow the upper lateral incisors in sequence, when the child is about ten years old, and the lower eye teeth (mandibular canines, cuspids) often appear at the same time.

The second premolars follow during the next year, then the upper canines. Usually, the second molars (twelve-year molars) come in at about the age of twelve years. The upper canines sometimes erupt with the second molars at about the same time, but in most instances, the canines' eruption precedes that of the molars by a matter of several months.

The third molars come in at about the age of seventeen years or later, and a considerable amount of jaw growth is needed after the age of twelve to allow room for these teeth. This growth often does not occur, and these third molars, or wisdom teeth, are often impacted or blocked into the jawbone, and are prevented from erupting by their position in the bone and the position of the teeth in front of them.

There is approximately an eighteen-month span of what can be considered normal in tooth eruption and every individual has his own individual pattern of eruption, his own sequence of eruption and his own dates of eruption which are normal for him. Although no specific ages for eruption of these teeth have been given, there are charts available with the average eruption dates (Appendix II).

Primary Dentition

The primary or deciduous dentition (or baby teeth) consists of eight incisors, two central and two lateral on the upper and on the lower arch, four canines (or eye teeth), and eight molars. The function of these teeth is the same as the function of their counterparts in the permanent dentition. However, these teeth are much smaller; the anatomy differs considerably; the enamel is much thinner; the teeth are much whiter; and the contours of the teeth are much more pronounced, especially at the gum line where they are much more convex. The dentin, as well as the enamel, is thinner; the pulp is larger; the roots, when they are present, are very widely spread; and in an X-ray the permanent teeth can be seen developing in crypts or follicles between the widely spread roots of the primary teeth.

The teeth begin to calcify (or to develop noticeably on X-rays) at about five months after conception. At eight months after conception the crowns of the incisors and the eye teeth and the first primary molars are largely formed. By birth, all the primary teeth have begun their formation. The noticeable radiographic formation of the permanent teeth begins at about six months of age. By the age of four the crowns of the central and lateral incisors, the cuspids and a portion of the crown of the bicuspids are formed. By the age of eight there will be radiographic evidence of the formation or presence of all of the permanent teeth.

The first tooth to appear is generally a central incisor, usually a lower incisor, although it may be an upper central incisor. The average age for the first tooth to appear is six months, although a child's first tooth may erupt as early as four months or as late as nine months. On rare occasions a child may be born with one already erupted.

The lateral incisors generally come in next, followed by the first primary molars. The canines will then erupt, and then the last teeth to make their appearance are the second molars. As is true for permanent dentition, each individual has his own pattern, order and dates of eruption of the primary teeth, although charts are available with average eruption dates (Appendix II). Generally by the age of two and one-half all of the primary teeth are in the mouth.

As stated earlier, it is easier to determine age from tooth eruption and development before the age of twelve years than it is after the age of twelve years. This is because the teeth in the jaw are in differing stages of development which can be seen on X-rays; there are more teeth involved; there are primary teeth still in the arch in the earlier years; and the dentist can assess the degree of calcification of the permanent teeth and the degree of dissolution of the roots of the primary teeth, pinpointing the age of a child under twelve within approximately three months. Once the twelve-year molars are in and all the permanent teeth have erupted, pinpointing the age becomes more difficult, although it can be generally done to within about an eighteen-month span, nine months on either side of the age.

Racial Variations

Although there are more variations of dentition within racial groups requiring consideration of other factors for proper deter-mination of race, there are general characteristics of the teeth and the facial bones which can provide some indication of the race of the subject.

In the Caucasian race, individuals usually have narrow, con-stricted arches, and the teeth tend to be of average size or on the small side of average, and tend to be crowded, especially on the front part of the dental arch.

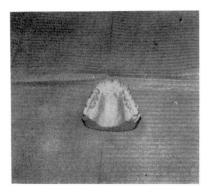

Figure 1. Cast of a typical Caucasian maxillary arch. Note the narrow, high palatal roof, relatively small teeth, and narrow arch form with crowding of the front teeth.

In the Negroid race, the dental arch tends to be broad and flat, and the palatal vault flat. The teeth tend to be larger than average and are often considerably larger than average. The arch length also tends to be longer than average, and may be much longer than average, and the upper and lower front teeth areas tend to be markedly protruded when viewed from the side.

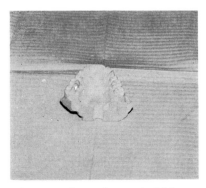

Figure 2. Cast of a typical Negro maxillary arch. Note the broad, relatively flat palatal roof, larger-than-average teeth, and broad, horseshoe-shaped arch with no anterior tooth crowding.

In the Mongoloid group, which includes Orientals, American Indians and Eskimos, the front teeth tend to be markedly shovel-shaped, that is, more concave on the tongue side with the tongue side bordered with heavy, round ridges, producing a shovel-shaped effect. There is also an anatomical landmark on the upper first permanent molar in all of the races, which in Mongoloids tends to be very pronounced and greatly enlarged (the Cusp of Carabelli). A further trait of Mongoloid individuals, which is present in a significant percentage of individuals and is not present in the other races, is the presence of a third root on the lower first permanent molar. The size of teeth among Mongoloid individuals tends to rank about average, and the arch length tends to be about average, although malocclusions (crooked teeth) are much less common than they are in Caucasians.

It should be remembered that all of these factors are complicated by intermarriage. The author has seen one case of shovel-shaped incisors and three-rooted lower molars in a Negro; on questioning, the Negro revealed that his great-grandmother was a full-blooded American Indian. So, although these racial characteristics are helpful in determination of the subject's race, these traits by themselves are not completely diagnostic of race but must be correlated with other factors provided by the medical pathologist.

JAW FUNCTION
Jaw Structure

The dental structure of a human being consists of an apparatus which resembles an upside down hammer and anvil. The anvil portion is the upper jawbone or maxillae. The fixed or anvil units of the biting mechanism are supported by many other bones of the skull, including some in the base of the skull. There are two maxilla, right and left, joined at the midline by a bony and fibrous fusion. Each maxilla is basically a boxlike bone with a hollowed out center called a sinus and four extensions that connect the maxilla with the cheek bone, the base of the skull, the bones of the nose and other bones of the front of the face. These maxillae are very thin and fragile structures and are meant to collapse on impact, protecting the other bones of the head and the bones of the base of the skull in much the same way as an energy-absorbing bumper is meant to protect an automobile.

The lower jaw, or mandible, is a single bone, unlike the upper jaw with its two maxillae. The lower jaw is a dense and heavy structure and resembles a bent horseshoe. It has a vertical portion, the ramus, which connects the mandible to the skull at a structure called the temporomandibular joint. The mandible also has a horizontal portion which runs parallel to the lower surface of the maxillae, for the most part ending at the chin.

The mandible contains no sinuses, but instead is made up of two layers. The outer layer is made up of heavy, thick, dense bone and is called the cortex. The inner layer is made up of bone marrow tissue and a network of smaller fibers of bone called the medulla, or spongy bone. The thin fibrules of bone in this spongy area are called trabeculae and are arranged along lines from the teeth through the main part of the jawbone into the vertical portion or ramus, and ending at the jaw joint areas. In such a way, the forces applied to the lower jawbone through the teeth are evenly distributed throughout the entire jawbone, and enough pressure or force is not allowed to build up at any one point to the degree that the jaw becomes fractured in normal use.

The joint that connects the upper and lower jaws is called the temporomandibular joint. This joint is probably the most flexible and the most unusual joint in the body. Unlike most other joints in the body, it contains a disc within the joint between the skull and the lower jawbone, dividing the joint into an upper and lower department, and it also contains cells, materials covering the bones, and numerous other components not found anywhere else in the body in the same combination. About the area of the jaw joints there are numerous muscles and ligaments which firmly but flexibly attach the lower jaw to the upper jaw and the base of the skull.

The temporomandibular joint, by its form and shape, not only has an influence on the way the teeth in the upper and lower jaw come together, but the positions of the teeth in the upper and lower jaws likewise influence and to some extent restrict the movements of this joint. Further, since there are two joints, a right and a left, these two joints acting together also restrict the movements of the lower jaw.

It can be seen that this joint is a very complex mechanism, and as such its exact nature and problems are beyond the scope of this book.

Jaw Movements

Although there are certain limitations to the movements of the lower jaw, within these limits the lower jaw is freely movable and there are many types of movements that the lower jaw is capable of making.

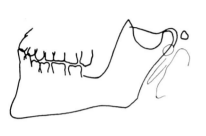
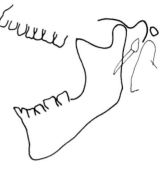

Figure 3.

Figures 3 and 4. Tracings from lateral head plate X-rays showing the jaw joint in its occlusal position (Figure 3); opened to its widest possible opening (Figure 3); opened as far as possible in a pure hinge movement (Figure 4); and in maximum protrusion (Figure 4). (Courtesy of Harry Sicher and Julius Tandler: *Anatomie für Zahnarzte*, Berlin, Springer, 1928.)

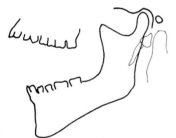
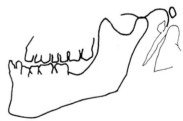

Figure 4.

There are two main types of movements that the jaw is capable of performing: those which are symmetrical and those which are nonsymmetrical. Symmetrical movements are those of protrusion or forward movement, retraction or backward movement, and the simple act of opening and closing. The protrusion and retraction movements are limited by the distance it is possible for the temporomandibular ligaments to stretch. The movements of opening and closing actually combine two types of movements, a pure hinge movement and a sliding movement. When the jaw begins to open, it first acts as a simple hinge, then once a point has been reached (approximately halfway) and the jaw continues to open wider, the jawbone itself begins to open physically forward with a sliding movement until it is open to the maximum. This combination of hinge movement and sliding movement in the opening and closing of jaws is found only in humans.

The nonsymmetrical movements the jaw is capable of making are lateral movements, or lateral swings to the right and to the left. Lateral swing movements are also limited by the amount of stretch possible in the temporomandibular ligaments.

The position of the jaws when all of the muscular apparatus is in a complete state of rest is called the rest position. In the rest position, the teeth are not in contact although the lips are. The rest position is unaffected by the presence or the absence of teeth or of their shape or the way in which they come together, but is determined instead by the tone of the muscles in the apparatus of the jaw. The rest position is important because if the teeth are positioned in such a way as to force the jaw to remain open to a degree greater than its rest position or if the teeth contain dental work such as crowns, bridges or other appliances which force the jaw open beyond its rest position, the muscles of the jaw go into spasm and over a period of time the result of all these factors may be distinctive damage both to the teeth and to the jaw joint itself.

Role of the Teeth

The movements of the jaw, whether retraction, protrusion, opening or closing, or lateral swings, are limited and modified by the teeth. The reverse is also true. The teeth are affected by the movements of which the jaw is capable. These relationships are known as occlusion. Occlusion refers to the relationship between the lower teeth and the upper teeth when they are in contact with each other. Another definition of occlusion could be the way in which the upper and lower teeth fit together in all working relationships of the lower and upper jaws. The movements and patterns of biting vary from individual to individual. Every individual has his own pattern of protrusion and retrusion, his own patterns of opening and closing and his own positions of lateral swing.

The teeth have a direct effect on the movements the jaw is capable of making during the biting process and are also capable of forcing the jaw into abnormal and damaging positions. The positions of the teeth can by themselves cause the lower jaw to slide away from its normal closing position into other abnormal positions, causing characteristic changes in the jaw joint itself.

These abnormal and damaging positions of the jaw likewise produce damage to the teeth themselves, some of which can be permanent and characteristic to the individual. Abnormal positions will cause facets or worn spots on the teeth. These change with age, but this change is very slow and occurs over a period of years and, for our purposes, they are characteristic and identifiable. If an individual bites an object capable of registering an impression of wear facets, a record will be left.

The position of the teeth is also affected by the way in which a person bites. If a tooth is lost, the teeth on either side will drift and close the space. The direction in which they drift and the degree to which they drift and the amount of closure of the space which occurs depends on the individual characteristics of the person's bite and can be influenced not only by the muscles of the jaw apparatus but by habits such as placing objects in the mouth, sucking on various objects, thrusting the tongue forward during the act of swallowing, or the simple projection of the tongue into a space where a tooth has been lost. Once a tooth has been lost, if the space is not filled with a bridge or a partial denture, then not only will the teeth on either side of the space drift into the space, but the tooth above the space will begin erupting again and will continue to erupt until it either contacts a lower tooth or contacts the lower gums. If it touches a portion of a lower tooth, it will tend to tip and rotate further into the space sideways until it again contacts either the other tooth or the gums.

All of these characteristics lead to specific individual differences in the position of teeth and wear facets on the teeth. All of these characteristics likewise have an effect on all of the movements it is possible for the jaw to make. Abnormal wear facets, areas of fractures on the teeth themselves, areas of abnormal or subnormal wear, spaces between the teeth, whether caused by loss of teeth or by disease processes, by habits or whether simply due to heredity, cause individual specific characteristic tooth positions and bite patterns, which likewise affect and are affected by the movements of the jaws.

Chapter 3 __ __ __ __ __ __ __ __ __

DENTAL EVIDENCE: SOURCES AND PROCEDURES

__ __ __ __ __ __ __ __ __ __ __ __

DENTAL EVIDENCE consists of human remains containing teeth, fragments of teeth or other oral structures, or of impressions of teeth (bite marks) in either human tissue or on objects left at the scene of the crime.

Dental records can lead to the identification of human remains when other, more conventional, means of identification cannot be used. The material from which these dental records are made consists of either unclaimed bodies with the dental records made from them at autopsy or afterwards, or of teeth or tooth fragments, or fragmentary remains of human oral tissues. These remains may be found accidentally or after a search in the field, or may be found by searching the area of a major disaster such as a fire, airline crash, train wreck or boating accident.

Bite marks may be found on any part of the body in a number of types of crimes to be described below, but they are most often found on the arms, legs, breasts, thighs, and on or about the head or neck. They are found also on items left at the scene of the crime such as apples or candy.

The usefulness of bite marks as evidence is based on the fact that no two people have the same bite marks, just as no two people have the same fingerprints. Although bite mark patterns (or bite registrations) do change very slowly over a period of years, they do not change over the normal length of time in which a criminal case will be investigated and prosecuted. Changes in the mouth and in the bite pattern, or the imprint left by the teeth when they close on an object, will only occur very slowly and over a period of many years. Then these changes are usually due to the loss of teeth by extraction, but there are always other characteristics in the dental arch which remain constant and from which identification of the maker of the bite mark can be determined. Characteristics such as diastemas (wide spaces between the teeth), crooked teeth, misplaced or rotated teeth, high eye teeth or extra teeth, and other unusual tooth alignments and arch forms do remain constant for the most part of life unless altered by extraction or orthodontic intervention (tooth straightening). Even in these later instances, though, there are enough differences in bite registrations which remain constant to make them valuable as evidence in the identification of assailants.

HUMAN REMAINS

The easiest dental identifications of unknown human remains come from intact jawbones with teeth; however, all fragments of jawbone, teeth and other portions of the oral structures should be carefully gathered and preserved because they can often provide trustworthy clues to identification. In cases where the entire dental arch or arches are present, but only a few teeth or tooth fragments can be found, this material is still of considerable value and can lead to an identification. From the specific gravity of individual teeth, it is possible for the dentist to determine the age of the individual. The presence of impacted teeth, extra teeth, missing teeth, and unusual position of teeth can be clues to identification of an individual when other means fail. In the case of human remains found in a fire, the color of the tooth fragments can indicate the temperature to which the individual was exposed and can aid in the determination of the cause of death, whether from exposure to heat, smoke inhalation, or other causes. The shape and outline of a dental arch may aid in identification, as can such factors as the presence of hereditary pitting in the enamel and changes in the enamel caused by medications such as tetracycline which produces a permanent yellowish stain that becomes a fluorescent, glowing orange under ultraviolet light. Discoloration can also be caused by high levels of fluoride. These high levels of fluoride are found only in certain areas of the country, and since it produces a distinctive brown-to-black stain on the teeth, the presence of such a stain can indicate that the victim is from one of those areas of the country. The use of dental records in particular can be a great aid in the

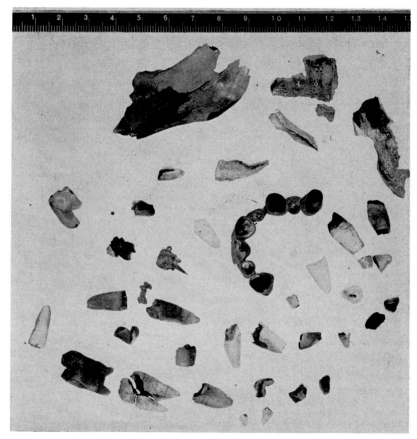

Figure 5. Sole remains of the victim of a house fire. The remains consisted of pieces of bone, teeth and dental restorations. (Courtesy of Gösta Gustafson: *Forensic Odontology*. New York, Elsevier, 1966, page 180; from Johanson Odontology faculty, Malmö, Sweden.)

identification of human remains. Dental charts are now generally used as an aid in identification, and their efficient use is described in Chapter 4.

Tooth fragments and jaw fragments will occasionally be found and may be presumed to be of human origin, but may not be. This can be determined by both careful anatomic observation by a dentist and, if necessary, a microscopic examination and evaluation. The structure of the bone supporting the tooth when viewed under a microscope is different for every species of animal, and a determination as to whether the remains are of human origin or of animal origin can be easily made by microscopic examination. Any questionable fragments of tooth or bones should be assumed to be of human origin until proven otherwise and should be collected in the manner described below and taken to the morgue for evaluation by the medical pathologist and by a dentist for an exact determination of their origin.

Individual Unidentified Remains

Human remains are sometimes found in fields, woods, floating in rivers, in solitary apartments, incinerated in the remains of automobiles, or almost anywhere.

Procedures

The following are procedures for police to follow in cases of individual unidentified remains in addition to the usual procedures:

1. The body will be carefully examined by the coroner or deputy coroner.
2. If the body is badly decomposed, the police officer should ask the coroner/deputy coroner if a dental identification should be requested, and if so, the police officer should notify the department dentist as described below.
3. If the body is not badly decomposed, the police officer should ask the coroner/deputy coroner to specifically examine not only for obvious wounds, but for any markings which could be construed as bite marks.
4. Any dental evidence present should be described in writing in a notebook.
5. Bite marks discovered at the scene should be photographed immediately.
6. When bite marks are noted by the coroner/deputy coroner, the police officer should ask for his permission to take impressions of the bite mark on the scene. If permission is declined for valid reason, the officer should remind the coroner that the dentist will wish to take impressions of the bite marks at autopsy.
7. The body should not be removed from the scene without the permission of the coroner/deputy coroner.
8. If a dental identification is requested by the coroner or his

deputy or if bite mark evidence is present, the officer should notify the department's dentist after the body is removed from the scene. The dentist should be given all information usually given consultants, according to each department's own usual procedures, but including the following information:

(a) type of case;

(b) circumstances surrounding the case;

(c) cause of death and condition of the body, (cause of death may be omitted if unknown);

(d) current location of body;

(e) if the request is for a dental identification or for evaluation of bite marks or other dental evidence;

(f) in bite mark cases, which photographs and impressions have been taken, and where they are being kept.

9. The dentist should be asked whether or not any laboratory work requiring a written work authorization will be necessary.

10. Police transportation should be offered the dentist.

11. Notations of the dental procedures performed should be made by the officer and photographs taken of these procedures at intervals.

12. Police should assist the dentist in assembling his equipment, if trained by the dentist.

13. If trained by the dentist, the police officer may assist in recording conditions present in the mouth.

14. If trained, the police officer may assist in some autopsy procedures.

15. The police officer, if trained and where state laws permit, should make any impressions requested by the dentist. Impressions should be taken to the laboratory where casts will be made from them.

16. Records should be transported to the place where they will be kept for evaluation by the dentist.

17. The police officer should interview in depth any potential relatives, if known, or when they appear, and as much information as possible about the victim should be obtained: clothes, jewelry, personal effects on or with him at the time,

condition of his teeth, and the name of the dentist(s) who treated him. If the person was in the military service, the branch of service, dates of service, and the time of separation, nature of his discharge, and the duty stations at which he served should be obtained; if the victim was ever in a mental institution or in a corrective institution, this information should be obtained because dental charts which could lead to identification may be still on file in the military records, or the records of the prison or mental institution.

18. If there is a clue as to which dentist(s) may have treated the person, the police officer should visit the dentist, obtain any dental records and X-rays the dentist may have on the victim, and bring them to the department dentist for evaluation.

19. If there are no leads as to which dentist may have treated the person in question, from the department dentist's examination it is often possible to determine the part of the country that the person was from, or the area of the country in which the dentist was trained to perform dental work. In these instances, copies of the dental chart, prepared by the police dentist, should be placed in professional journals in those parts of the country and sent to the dentists in the area of the crime or where the body was found who were trained in those areas of the country. The dentist will have a book called the American Dental Directory, which will have this information in it. In cases of no clues at all, the chart will be placed in the Journal of the American Dental Association. Usually the dentist will place the chart in the journals and send them to other dentists, but sometimes he will ask the police officer to so do, in which case he will provide names, addresses and all other details.

20. When charts begin to come in from other parts of the country, the trained police officer may perform a general screening of the charts; he should collect those which would appear to be the most obvious matches and put them together. In no case, however, should the officer withhold any incoming charts from the dentist. To do so, or to do any screening of a more extensive nature would consist of practicing dental diagnosis, and this may only be done by the dentist.

21. All records received should be photocopied and placed in the department files for future reference before the originals are returned to the dentist who sent them.

22. Occasionally, where death is due to gunshot or where the body is badly decomposed, portions of the dental structure may be missing. In this case, the police officer may be dispatched to the recovery site to search for any additional fragments of bone or teeth. If found there, they should be placed in an appropriately sized plastic container containing 10% formalin. The fragments should be brought back to the morgue for examination by the dentist and pathologist.

Major Disasters

In the case of a major disaster, the area around the disaster site should be searched very carefully for human remains. Preferably this should be done by a team or an identification committee (disaster squad), consisting of one or more medical pathologists, one or more dentists, and a number of police officers and evidence technicians. The organization of such a squad is beyond the scope of this book; see the bibliography for a source if more information on this subject is desired.

Procedures

Following are procedures the police should follow in mass disasters in addition to the usual procedures associated with the investigation of such cases. The details of what information to give the dentist when he is called in on the case are not included because in mass disasters it will not be the police officer, but a federal official most likely from the FBI or the Department of Transportation, who will summon the dentist or the members of the state or regional dental identification squad. This official will give all necessary and pertinent information to the dentist(s) when they arrive. However, the police may be asked to provide transportation for the dentist(s) from their location to the scene.

1. Working in cooperation with officials of the medical examiner or coroner's office, and possibly with officials of the FBI, the entire area where the catastrophe occurred should be carefully searched for any fragments or remains of human tissues or structures. When found, these fragments should be carefully collected.

2. Fragments should be placed in bottles containing 10% formalin.

3. Material, when collected, should be taken to the morgue. In most instances of mass disaster there will be an emergency morgue set up at a nearby hospital where the dentists and pathologists and officials of the FBI will attempt to make identifications. Since the FBI identification team works entirely on the basis of fingerprints and thus will be dealing with the hands, their work will not interfere with the work of the police dentist(s) if a dental emergency team has been employed.

4. When dental identifications are called for, the dentist(s) will make a chart for each individual in question and will probably take X-rays. If trained by the dentist, the police officer may assist in preparing the chart notations.

5. Where commercial carriers are involved, representatives of the carrier should be contacted and a passenger list obtained.

6. Very detailed interviews should be conducted by the police officer with relatives of the victim, and as much information as possible about the victim should be obtained from them, as described in Item 17 in the previous section dealing with the handling of individual unidentified remains.

7. The family dentist(s) of the victim, if known, should be contacted and questioned in detail and records obtained, by subpoena if necessary, for evaluation and comparison with the records constructed by the forensic dentist, and for comparison with the remains. In addition to individual dental records, any and all X-rays, study models and notes should be obtained in the same manner. Furthermore, in addition to the individual dentist's records, any dental records in existence in the military, mental hospitals, prisons, or any institutions should be obtained, by subpoena if necessary.

8. Occasional problems may arise from the fact that there may be mistakes in the family dentist's own charting on record cards. This occurs generally in instances where the charting is not done by the dentist, but by a dental assistant who may or may not be experienced in charting. Where these cases of doubt

occur, the dentist should be called in to view the victim or portions of the remains at the mortuary or morgue. In many cases the dentist will recognize his own work. In cases where the dentist does not recognize his own work, further comparison with other dental records from other sources as described above may combine to provide a definitive identification.

BITE MARKS

Bite marks may be found on any part of the body in a number of types of crimes, most often on the arms, legs, breasts, thighs, and about the head or neck. It is important, if the subject is alive, to question him carefully as to whether or not he (or she) recalls being bitten. Because the bite mark, which may be useful as primary or as supportive evidence, may be present on any part of the body and not necessarily the area in which the primary injury occurred, the entire person should be examined for the presence of bite marks, either by the physician in the hospital or by the medical pathologist at autopsy.

The most important factors in determining the usefulness of a bite mark as criminal evidence are these: The bite must be hard enough to significantly damage the underlying tissues or to inflict a row of puncture wounds; and the bite mark must be found and a permanent record made of its appearance as soon as possible before the body's repair processes or the degenerative processes after death alter or obliterate the mark. Investigators in Sweden have found that a bite mark may, in a live individual, remain visible for from four to thirty-six hours; in a deceased individual, from twelve to twenty-four hours after death, depending upon the amount of damage inflicted by the bite and upon the part of the body on which the bite has been inflicted.

Methods of handling the bite mark evidence are described categorically by crime below. Preserving evidence of the bite mark is only half the job of identification of the assailant, however; the bite marks must be traced to the teeth of the suspect. Procedures for preparing materials for comparison with the victim's bite mark are indicated below. Sometimes the cases are reversed: the victim has bitten the assailant; in those cases, the procedures should be reversed by merely substituting "victim" for "suspect" and vice versa.

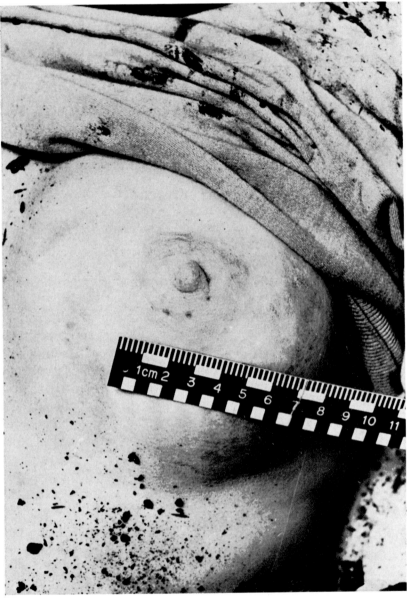

Figure 6. A murder victim with bite marks on the breast. (Courtesy of Gösta Gustafson: *Forensic Odontology*, New York, Elsevier, 1966, page 142; from Ström, personal communication, 1963c.)

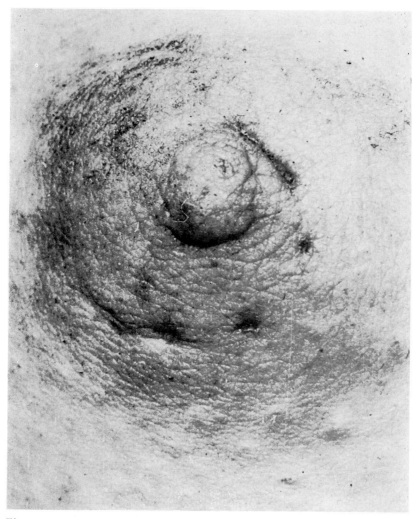

Figure 7. Closeup of the bite marks in Figure 6 showing the long imprints of the upper front teeth at the upper right and the pointed impressions of the lower front teeth at the lower left. Note the spaces between the tooth prints, which, along with the tooth alignment shown by the marks, are characteristic of the person who inflicted this bite. (Courtesy of Gösta Gustafson: *Forensic Odontology.* New York, Elsevier, 1966, page 143; from Ström, personal communication 1963c.)

It is important in evaluating some cases to differentiate human bite marks from animal bite marks. This is easily done since the

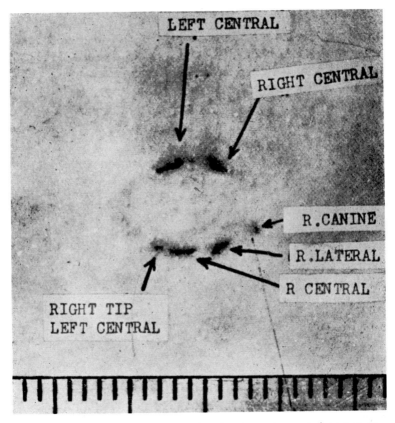

Figure 8. Photograph of a bite mark showing how the teeth which inflicted the tooth prints can be identified by the type of mark they leave. (Courtesy of Gösta Gustafson: *Forensic Odontology.* New York, Elsevier, 1966, page 153; from Simpson 1951.)

dental arch of animals is much narrower than it is in humans. Animal teeth are generally much sharper and the indentations smaller and deeper. In human bites, the outline of the arch is more U-shaped, broader, and the indentations of the teeth are broader, and shallower and more blunt in appearance. Bite marks inflicted by horses are considerably wider and much more U-shaped than human bites, and the indentations made by the teeth are approximately twice the width of marks made by human teeth. If there is any question as to whether a bite mark has been inflicted by a human or by an animal, the photographs, impressions and descrip-

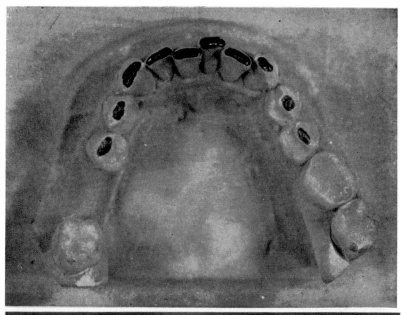

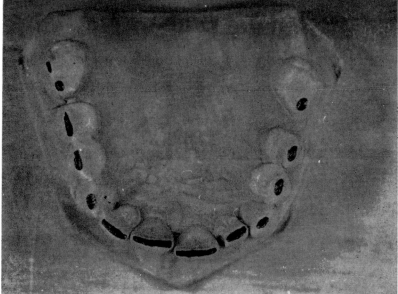

Figure 9. Casts of the teeth of a suspect in a case where dental evidence was found. The teeth are marked for comparison with an impression of the bite mark found on the victim. Courtesy of Gösta Gustafson: *Forensic Odontology*, New York, Elsevier, 1966, page 151.

tions indicated for a human bite should be made and the material presented to the dentist for evaluation and possible elimination.

Assault and Battery

Victims of beatings occasionally are found bearing bite marks. These bite marks are generally on the head, neck or on the forearm, and consist of a double semicircular line of indentations with which bleeding may or may not be associated. These bite marks are sometimes difficult to find because they are associated with other injuries such as bruises or cuts due to the object or objects with which the beating was administered.

It goes without saying that when a person is attacked, that per-

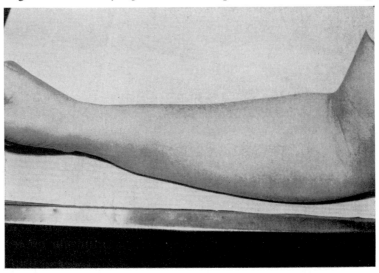

Figure 10. Bite mark on the forearm.

son will attempt to defend himself by any means possible. Therefore, this is one of the types of cases in which the assailant, if he is apprehended within four to thirty-six hours, may be found to have bite marks on his person which can be matched with the teeth of his victim. These bite marks are generally on the hands and arms or about the head and neck, and may be associated with injuries such as bruises, cuts or scratches.

Battery is one case where it is sometimes necessary to differentiate human bite marks from animal bite marks in the manner indicated previously.

Procedures

When a bite mark is found on a battery victim, the following procedures should be followed:

1. A detailed written description of the bite mark's appearance should be made by the investigating officer.

2. A saliva smear should be taken by moistening a large cotton roll in sterile distilled water and wiping it gently over the area about the bite mark several times. The cotton ball should be placed in a sterile test tube or wide-mouthed jar and sealed, to be examined later in the laboratory for traces of saliva from which the blood type of the assailant may be determined.

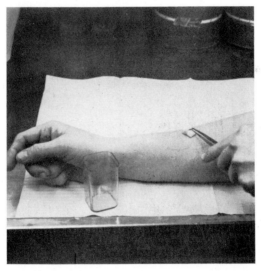

Figure 11. Saliva wash being made of a bite mark.

3. Color and black-and-white photographs should be taken in detail and from every angle. A millimeter ruler should be placed beside or under the mark to record the size of the mark. Additional photographs using different lighting and shading effects, or with red or blue filters or with infrared film may be desired.

4. After obtaining the victim's consent, impressions should be taken using rubber base or silicone materials with a custom

Dental Evidence

tray technique described in Chapter 8. The impressions should be sent to a laboratory where they will be poured up in dental stone.

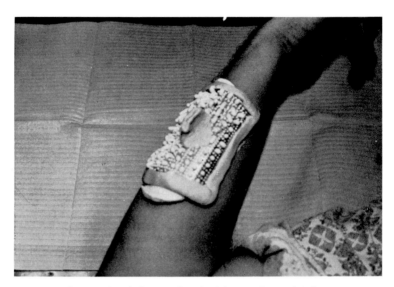

Figure 12. Impression being made of a bite mark on the forearm.

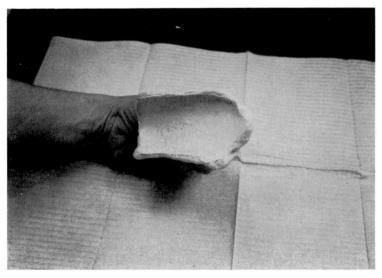

Figure 13. Finished alginate hydrocolloid impression of a bite mark.

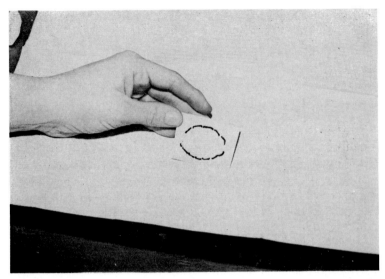

Figure 14. Stone cast of the bite mark in Figure 13, with tooth positions carefully marked for later comparison with casts of a suspect's teeth.

5. The impressions, photographs and all other records should then be taken to the dentist for evaluation.

Child Abuse

Child abuse is one area in which dental evidence is especially common. Children who are beaten by their parents, babysitters or older brothers and sisters or relatives are often bitten as part of their torture, and these bite marks are generally found on the upper arms and about the head and on the upper torso. These bite marks seem proportionately larger than a bite mark on an adult due to the small size of the child.

Bite marks on the battered child may be associated with and partially masked by other injuries, such as bruises and cuts, and a careful examination of the entire body of the child is essential. Since many hospitals do not as a matter of general procedure examine suspected cases of child abuse for the presence of bite marks, the police officer called to the hospital should as a matter of routine in all instances ask the doctor examining the child to specifically look for bite marks or any bruises or other indentations which could be inflicted by teeth.

Bite mark evidence in the child abuse syndrome is of more value in determining the identity of the child's attacker rather than proving the fact of child abuse, as other injuries are generally present; but in questionable cases where the injuries are relatively minor and where the parent claims the injuries were due to a fall or accident, the presence of bite marks on the child can be considered as presumptive evidence of abuse, regardless of what the parent says.

Procedures

When bite marks are found on a child in association with suspected child abuse, the following procedures should be followed:

1. A written description of the bite mark should be made by the police officer who handles the complaint and should also be requested from the doctor who examines the child.

2. A saliva smear should be taken as described in the section on procedures for handling assault and battery cases (Item 2).

3. Photographs in color and black-and-white should be taken from every conceivable angle using techniques of lighting and shading to emphasize details of the bite marks. A millimeter ruler should be placed beside or under the mark to give a record of the size of the mark. Photographs using filters and infrared photographs may be indicated as described in Chapter 5.

4. With the prior approval of the child's examining medical doctor and the approval of the child's parents and after an explanation of the reason for this procedure has been made, an impression should be made of the bite marks using a silicone or rubber base material and a custom tray technique described in Chapters 7 and 8. The impression will then be taken to a laboratory where a cast will be made of the impression in dental stone.

5. The casts, photographs and all other records pertaining to the bite should be taken to a dentist for evaluation.

Sex Crimes

Bite marks are frequently associated with sex crimes. These marks are found about the head and neck, or on or about the breasts, forearms, thighs or abdomen, and look like either a row of indentations with which bleeding may or may not be associated, or may look like raised blue or red-blue circular bruises. Bruises caused by a predominant sucking action, in contrast to a biting action, appear more or less almond shaped with pointed or slightly rounded ends, are much narrower than a normal bite mark, and the entire area is discolored. Although a sucking action involves some biting force due to the nature of this action, the biting force is rarely enough to produce a bite mark which may be recorded and used with any degree of validity, although borderline cases do occur.

In cases of sex crimes, as well as other types of assaults, the victims will occasionally bite their assailants in an attempt to defend themselves, and any suspect arrested in connection with this type of crime within thirty-six hours should be examined by a medical doctor or by a medical doctor and a dentist for the presence of bite marks which could match the bite registration and impressions of the victim's teeth.

Procedures

When bite marks are found in association with sex crimes, the following procedures should be performed.

1. A detailed written description should be made of the bite marks by the officer and by the examining medical doctor.
2. A saliva smear or wash should be taken of the area as described in the section on procedures for handling assault and battery cases (Item 2).
3. Photographs in color and black-and-white should be made of the mark with a millimeter ruler placed beneath the bite mark to provide a record of the size of the mark.
4. After obtaining consent from the victim and explaining the purpose of this procedure, impressions should be made of the victim's teeth and the victim's bite registration obtained, using techniques described in Chapter 7. These will provide records which can be used for comparison with bite marks which may be found on suspects. A cast should then be made of the impressions at a laboratory.
5. The casts, photographs and all other records of the bite marks of the victim and/or suspect should be taken to a dentist for evaluation.

Homicides

Bite marks are occasionally found in cases of homicide. They are most often found in homicides associated with child abuse and with sex crimes. In these cases, bite marks are most commonly found on the upper torso, the neck, the forearms and the thighs. The appearance of the bite marks will be similar to those described previously. It is important that the police specifically request that the forensic pathologists at the coroner's office examine the entire body for bites before proceeding with the autopsy and not limit their observations to the area of the body around the primary site of injury.

Procedures

In recording bite marks on homicide cases at autopsy, the following procedures should be followed:

1. A detailed written description of the bite marks should be made by the officer at the scene, and by the medical pathologist at autopsy.
2. A saliva smear should be taken of the area of the bite mark, as described in the section on procedures for handling assault and battery cases (Item 2).
3. Black-and-white and color photographs should be taken at the scene if the bite mark is found then. If the bite mark is discovered at autopsy, black-and-white and color photographs should be taken using a millimeter ruler placed next to the bite mark to indicate the size of the mark.
4. Impressions should be taken of the bite mark in rubber base or silicone rubber base impression material using a custom tray and techniques described in Chapter 7. Casts of the impressions should be made at a laboratory.
5. All casts, photographs, and other materials pertaining to the bite mark(s) should be taken to a dentist for evaluation.

Physical Evidence

Items of physical evidence found at or near the scene of a crime often contain bite marks, saliva or in a few instances, pieces of teeth. Examples of such physical evidence are food, such as fruit; vegetables like pickles, cucumbers, carrots or other large, firm vegetables; pieces of cheese; sausage or other types of large luncheon meat; chewing gum; cigar remnants; cigarette filters; bottle caps and wooden or plastic objects with which a person could strike another.

When confronted with physical evidence which came into contact with the teeth or mouth, the officer, of necessity, must decide which of three ways it must be handled: whether it needs to be tested for saliva, whether a bite mark needs to be preserved, or whether tests of a tooth fragment need to be made. It is necessary to make a choice between preservation of a bite mark and testing for blood type through saliva sampling because the one procedure eliminates the possibility of the other procedure. If there is any doubt, a dentist should be called immediately.

Bite marks are often found on all the items listed above except the last two. On bottle caps, the mark is likely to be a scratch mark. On the other items a bite mark is often found of which an impression and cast can be made. In all cases where it appears there is a bite mark, preservation of this evidence takes precedence over preservation of a saliva sample.

In some cases, the bite mark is not clear enough to make an identification through its preservation. In these cases, the items should be tested for saliva. Examples of items which usually have bite marks too poor for use are chewing gum, cigar remnants, and cigarette filters. In particular, chewing gum, although there may be bite marks, is less valuable for bite marks than for saliva because chewing gum adheres to portions of the teeth and leaves roughened or blurred areas, thus compromising the accuracy of the registration of the tooth impression. In addition, if an object is badly mutilated and does not contain any clear bite impression which can be identified, the object can and should be tested for saliva, regardless of the category or type of object it is, whether fruit, vegetable, meat or another substance.

Although traces of saliva are found on all the types of physical evidence described except wooden or plastic objects used for striking, it is important not to test any of the items containing a bite mark for saliva because the value of the bite mark evidence or tooth impression contained in them will be destroyed by testing them for saliva. The distilled water used to dissolve the saliva from the article will also dissolve, erode, or otherwise modify the surface of the object being tested, obliterating the bite mark; while knowing the blood group from the saliva test is valuable in the area of supportive evidence, it cannot in itself identify the individual where the bite mark can, if it is clear.

Finally, it occasionally occurs that a wooden or a plastic object is used to strike an individual in the face and pieces of tooth structure break off and become imbedded in the object. When the object with the fragments is found, these fragments can be subjected to chemical analysis in the laboratory and matched with samples of the victim's tooth and can then identify the weapon used, or if wielded by the person attacked, can identify the attacker. It is not necessary to test the possible weapon for saliva traces, because no significant amounts of saliva will become imbedded in or on the object to provide a positive test.

Procedures

When a small piece of physical evidence, as described above, is found and it is felt necessary by the officer or the dentist following the guidelines just described to test the item for saliva, the following procedures should be followed:

1. The item should be carefully picked up and placed in a test tube, bottle or other container with enough sterile distilled water to completely cover the object. The container is then completely closed and sealed.
2. The outside of the container is marked with the name of the object, the type of case, and any other details necessary according to the usual procedures of each police jurisdiction.
3. The material is then sent to a laboratory where the distilled water will be tested for saliva traces and blood grouping.

When a small item of physical evidence is found and it has been determined according to the guidelines that the item must be considered for bite mark evidence, the following procedures should be followed:

1. A complete written description should be made.
2. Black-and-white and color photographs should be taken, with lighting to emphasize details of the impression, using a millimeter ruler to indicate size.
3. Impressions should be made of the marks, using either rubber base material, silicone rubber base impression material, or alginate impression material; these impressions should be taken

immediately to prevent the likelihood of alteration, modification or destruction of the bite mark through decomposition or through the adverse effects of temperature changes. The impression should be taken to a laboratory to have a cast poured in dental stone.

4. The suspect's bite mark in a similar object should be subjected to examination and comparison with the marks left on the original object or a cast of it under a binocular comparison microscope, as described in Appendix I.

When a tooth fragment is found imbedded in a wooden or plastic object, the following procedures should be performed:

1. The object should be examined for other types of evidence, such as fingerprints, and all other procedures should be done first before the dental evidence is gleaned; care should be taken that the other evidence is not disturbed or damaged.

2. A dentist should be called to make filings of the tooth. The tooth must remain in the object to be shown to the jury, and only a dentist will be able to remove small portions of the tooth skillfully enough not to damage the usefulness of the evidence left in the object.

3. The filings should be placed in a clean glass container and stored until a suspect is apprehended if it is thought to be the assailant's tooth; it may be tested immediately if thought to be the victim's tooth.

4. The dentist will specify which tests (for mineral content, for example) will be taken and which laboratory will be used. The police should then take the samples to the laboratory along with a work order prepared by the dentist. The police officer should pick up the material and results when finished and return the results to the dentist and take the filings to a storage place.

Evidence from Suspect

When a suspect is apprehended and a case in which bite mark evidence, except physical evidence, is present, the following procedures should be followed:

1. He should be asked to give his permission for the procedures below; he should be told why they are necessary and reminded that they could possibly clear him; if he refuses per-

mission, a court order or a search warrant should be obtained for impressions and casts of his mouth and for his bite registration.

2. In cases where a saliva sample from the victim's bite mark showed the presence of blood groups, a blood sample should be taken for blood group determination by medical personnel.

3. Impressions should be made of his teeth using an alginate material; detailed techniques for this and the next two procedures will follow in Chapters 7 and 8.

4. A custom tray should be made and secondary impressions should be made of his teeth with a rubber base or a silicone rubber base impression material.

5. A bite registration should be obtained by having the suspect bite into a wafer of metal-impregnated wax.

6. All materials should be compiled and taken to the dentist for evaluation.

When a suspect is apprehended and a case in which dental physical evidence is present, the following procedures should be performed:

1. The suspect should be asked to give his permission for the necessary procedures. He should be told why they are necessary and reminded that they could possibly clear him; if he refuses permission, a court order or a search warrant should be obtained for the procedures.

2. In cases where the evidence was tested for saliva, and it showed the presence of a blood group, a blood sample should be taken for blood group determination.

3. In cases where the evidence was of a bite mark, the suspect should bite into a material identical or similar to the original material. If this is not practical, bite registration wax should be used.

4. The sample of the suspect's bite mark in wax or other material should be compared under the binocular comparison microscope by the technician with the original physical evidence or cast of that evidence as described in Appendix I.

5. In cases where the evidence was a tooth fragment imbedded in an object, a dentist should be called to obtain filings of the suspect's teeth; the filings should be taken by the police along

with a work order to the laboratory chosen by the dentist, and picked up along with the written results when the test has been completed.

6. All material should be compiled and taken to the dentist for evaluation.

Chapter 4 ____ __ ___ __ __ __ __ __ __ __

DENTAL RECORDS

__ __ __ ___ __ __ __ __ __ __ __ __

Dental records are being used by police departments and coroner's offices as a means of identification of badly decomposed, severely burned, or otherwise mutilated human remains so that identification by the conventional means cannot be accomplished. Identification by dental records is useful in mass disasters, airline crashes, disasters at sea, and instances when the body has been submerged for great periods of time and the facial features have been changed beyond recognition. Police officials should know that occasionally the only means by which an identification can be arrived at is through the use of good dental records.

When assistance in making an identification from dental records is desired, a dentist should be retained either by the police department or by the coroner's office and asked to make a detailed chart of the victim's mouth. The police department and coroner's office should have on hand suitable charts for the dentist's use; acceptable and desired charts are described below.

The chart should be filled out by the dentist in a careful and precise manner, correlating his findings with X-rays and a thorough examination of the supporting tissues and the general oral environment. When the charting is done carefully and precisely the result is a legal document capable of withstanding the scrutiny of the courts and of providing the dentists to whom the chart is sent directly or who see it in the journals with an accurate instrument with which to compare their own charts.

The police officer and evidence technician should not in any way make a dental chart for any individual, deceased or alive. This kind of work may, under the law, be done only by a dentist. Still, however, the police officer and the evidence technician should know what a dental chart looks like, what variations are common and

48

acceptable, and how to read a dental chart. If the police officer and evidence technician know what elements go into a dental chart and are aware of the common and accepted variations and can read them, it is obvious that they can be more effective partners with the dentist who makes the identifications in much the same way a dental assistant or a dental laboratory technician is a more effective partner with the dentist if he or she is able to read a dental chart and is not competent if he or she cannot do so. Although the police officer and the evidence technician may not themselves prepare a dental chart, the officer, in addition to knowing how to read a chart, should be prepared to assist the dentist in marking the chart as the dentist makes the examination if the dentist so trains the police officer or technician; to assist the dentist in contacting the practitioners in the area from which it is felt the victim comes to enlist their assistance in obtaining possible matching dental charts; to see that all of the proper material is gathered for the dentist to evaluate; and to aid in this evaluation by compiling the charts by common characteristics as they come in. The final process of elimination and any definitive judgments made relating to dental identification must, however, be left to the dentist.

Types of Charts

There are many types of dental charts available, and all have certain characteristics in common. All may be used or can be adapted for dental evidence work. Some, however, are better than others. All have images representing the teeth, and all have some place on the images to mark the types of tooth decay and other forms of mouth illnesses present. All charts should have some blank spaces beneath the symbols representing the teeth in which one can write a short description of each tooth. All charts should also have on them a place to write other pertinent information concerning the case. Charts are available from a number of commercial companies; however, a police department or coroner's office can design its own charts with the aid of a dentist at less cost.

One type of dental chart for forensic use has images representing both the primary and permanent teeth. Both the crowns and roots are shown so that any unusual patterns in bone development or bone resorption due to various disease processes which can occur in the mouth, abnormal roots, and various types of root canal fillings and

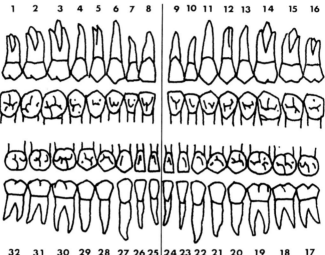

FORM A

Coroner's number _____ Police case number _____

Name of examining pathologist _____ Police dept. _____

Name of senior investigating officer _____

Date of dental examination _____

Location of dental examination _____

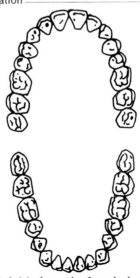

Adult's forensic dental chart.

FORM B

ADULT

		CHILD
1		
2		A
3		B
4		C
5		D
6		E
7		F
8		G
9		H
10		I
11		J
12		K
13		L
14		M
15		N
16		O
17		P
18		Q
19		R
20		S
21		T
22		
23		
24		
25		Observations:
26		
27		
28		
29		
30		
31		Observations:
32		

FORM A

Coroner's number _____ Police case number _____

Name of examining pathologist _____ Police dept. _____

Name of senior investigating officer _____

Date of dental examination _____

Location of dental examination _____

Child's forensic dental chart.

FORM B

ADULT

CHILD

ADULT		CHILD	
1	_____	A	_____
2	_____	B	_____
3	_____	C	_____
4	_____	D	_____
5	_____	E	_____
6	_____	F	_____
7	_____	G	_____
8	_____	H	_____
9	_____	I	_____
10	_____	J	_____
11	_____	K	_____
12	_____	L	_____
13	_____	M	_____
14	_____	N	_____
15	_____	O	_____
16	_____	P	_____
17	_____	Q	_____
18	_____	R	_____
19	_____	S	_____
20	_____	T	_____
21	_____		
22	_____		
23	_____		
24	_____		
25	_____	Observations:	
26	_____		
27	_____		
28	_____		
29	_____		
30	_____		
31	_____	Observations:	
32	_____		

FORM A

Coroner's number ——————————— Police case number ——————————

Name of examining pathologist ——————————— Police dept. ———————————

Name of senior investigating officer ————————————————————————————————

Date of dental examination ——

Location of dental examination ————————————————————————————————————

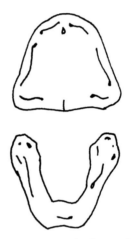

Edentulous forensic dental chart.

FORM B

ADULT		CHILD
1 _____		A _____
2 _____		B _____
3 _____		C _____
4 _____		D _____
5 _____		E _____
6 _____		F _____
7 _____		G _____
8 _____		H _____
9 _____		I _____
10 _____		J _____
11 _____		K _____
12 _____		L _____
13 _____		M _____
14 _____		N _____
15 _____		O _____
16 _____		P _____
17 _____		Q _____
18 _____		R _____
19 _____		S _____
20 _____		T _____
21 _____		
22 _____		
23 _____		
24 _____		
25 _____		Observations:
26 _____		
27 _____		
28 _____		
29 _____		
30 _____		
31 _____		Observations:
32 _____		

past evidence of jaw surgery such as apicoectomies (surgical removal of the end of the tooth root), can be shown when present.

Another acceptable chart contains patterns of circles, one circle inside another with the entire pattern divided into quarters. Each of these patterns represents a tooth, with one of these patterns on a chart to represent each of the permanent teeth and each of the primary teeth. These circular patterns may be arranged either in a semicircle or on a straight line. The uppers and the lowers will be delineated, and the right and left will be designated. Below each circle pattern will be a number and a letter identifying the tooth. Adult teeth will be numbered from 1 to 32, and the primary teeth will be identified by the letters A thru T. At the top of the chart will be space for information concerning the case, and at the bottom of the chart will be a list of numbers from 1 to 32 and letters from A to T, at the side of which the dentist can write the actual disease condition of each tooth present.

A configuration which should be either included on the chosen chart or available as a second chart, should the dentist desire it, has a picture of the teeth lined up on an ideal arch form. On this it is possible to show whether or not the tooth is in an abnormal position, i.e. whether or not the tooth is positioned toward the cheek or toward the tongue, whether it is lapped, rotated or completely out of line or separated from the other teeth by spaces. Thus it is possible to show the abnormal positions, spaces and malocclusions which could be characteristic of the individual and can aid in obtaining an identification.

Another useful type of chart which should be on hand shows a picture of the upper and lower jaws without any teeth (an edentulous arch). Although there are ridges on the roof of the mouth, it has been shown that these ridges change enough with time so that they cannot be relied upon to make a positive identification. However, marks are sometimes made on the gums by dentures and unusual types of false teeth. This can be designated on this type of chart, and the presence of any abnormal conditions of the gums, any growths and tumors, and any submerged roots or other types of pathology which could be used to identify the individual without teeth can also be shown on this type of chart.

A final type of chart which should be available contains a skeletal profile consisting of a profile outline of the face with the eyes and the upper and lower front teeth set into the outline of the upper and lower jawbones, upon which the dentist can chart cephalometric findings (bone growth pattern tracings), when indicated. This may be occasionally useful in the identification of teenagers or smaller children.

Dr. Gösta Gustofson, in Sweden, has recommended a type of

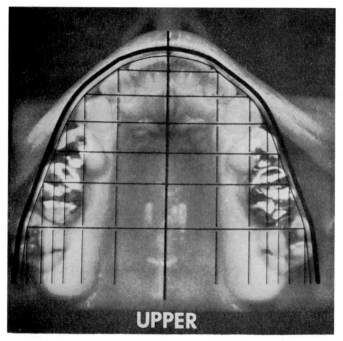

Figure 18. Photograph of dental arch superimposed on a grid. This can be used as a substitute for a conventional ante mortem dental chart. (Courtesy of Unitek Corporation, Monrovia, California.)

chart which consists of a composite color photograph with a closeup front view of the head and neck, with pictures of the upper and lower teeth below this, and a written description of all the dental work in the mouth written below that. Until recently, this type of photographic record was difficult and expensive to prepare, but cameras have been recently developed which will take these types of photographs quickly and inexpensively. Photographic records of this type are highly desirable for companies whose employees and

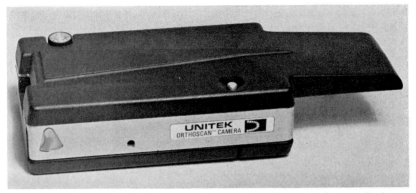

Figure 19. The Unitek Orthoscan Camera is used to take intraoral photographs for dental records such as the photograph in Figure 18. (Courtesy of Unitek Corporation, Monrovia, California.)

staff are exposed to a lot of travel or are in high risk situations, are especially suited for airlines, the military services, the merchant marine, the police and other regulatory agencies, and could easily be routinely taken along with the traditional mug shot when criminals are held in detention.

In the future it is possible that Dr. Gustofson's concept of charting could, with sufficient interest and money allocated to the project, be extended in such a way as to make the cumbersome job of placing charts in journals and contacting individual dentists at least partially, if not completely, obsolete. It is possible as a part of the routine processing of criminals to take pictures of the upper and lower teeth at the time they are processed for admission into the city or county prison. These photographs could then be classified by the dentist in any one of a number of ways based either on the pattern of teeth lost, numbers of teeth lost, or on the presence or absence or condition (filled or unfilled) of the bicuspids, or indeed, by all of these methods. The composite photographs of the frontal view of the face with the upper and lower arches and with the written description beneath it of the restorations and conditions of each tooth could then be committed to microfilm.

Further, the entire system could then be keyed into a computer and cross-indexed by each of the ways in which the dental condition was classified by the dentist on the basis of absence of teeth, pattern of missing teeth, absence or presence of bicuspids and their conditions, whether filled or unfilled. This would revolutionize the field of dental identification, since the computer would be able, in a matter of a short time, to select anywhere from a dozen to several hundred possible dental reference photographs, eliminating all others, greatly expediting the process of dental identification, and eliminating the traditional weak spot in the field of dental evidence, the occasional inability of the private dentist to locate in his own files a dental chart which fits the description on the police chart reasonably well. The potential for this is approximately as great, in this author's opinion, as the potential was for the field of human fingerprinting fifty years ago.

Systems of Charting

The properly filled out chart prepared by the dentist will clearly and accurately record all conditions in the mouth in a way that they can be easily recognized and identified. Any missing teeth should be completely blocked out. Any teeth which are filled should have a filling drawn in just the way it appears in the mouth. Any teeth replaced by a bridge or partial denture should have that bridge or partial denture indicated on the chart. Any teeth which have undergone any nerve treatments or any nerve canal treatments associated with surgery should be noted on the chart. Any unfilled cavities present should also be marked on the chart just as they appear in the mouth. Any teeth which are unerupted or impacted (blocked and prevented from erupting hence still in the jawbones), should be marked and represented on the chart. Any unusual type of dental work or any oral disease conditions should be noted on the chart; for example, occasionally a spade or star will be carved out of a cap on a front tooth, and this should be noted because such a thing will obviously be an identifying mark.

The conditions indicated on the chart are consistent from one dentist to another, but the methods by which the facts are indicated often vary according to the preference of the dentist, but then the dentist will be consistent in his variation of the method or system. It is acceptable, for instance, to indicate missing teeth with an "X" or a slash instead of completely shading the tooth out, as long as the dentist is completely consistent in his use of this symbol, as almost all are. Some types of charts (the circle within the circle divided into quarters) do not allow drawing the restoration as it appears in the mouth, but only coloring in the surfaces or sides of the tooth where decay is present. In situations such as these, on the bottom of the chart there should be a written explanation consisting of the tooth's number and a written description of the type of restoration, crown, bridge or filling present in the tooth, or the general condition otherwise. If this is done, this type of chart is also acceptable.

The importance of dental charting done in a consistent, accurate and thorough manner is illustrated by the following case history. On September 31, 1934, in Albury, Australia, the remains of a young girl wearing pajamas and a towel around her head was found burned beyond recognition inside a gunny sack in the basement of a building. There were no clues either to the identity of the victim or to the perpetrator's motives. Due to the peculiar circumstances, it was presumed that the case was a homicide and that the girl had been transported to this site, as there was no evidence of a fire anywhere in the vicinity.

In an attempt to obtain the identity of the girl, impressions were made of her teeth and casts were made from the impressions. Photographs were made of the cast, but not the teeth, and a dental chart was prepared and copies of it circulated among the dentists in Australia. Although a number of charts with possible matches were sent to the police, there were no positive results for ten years.

In May, 1944 police received a tip that the remains could be those of Linda Agostini, missing since the autumn of 1934. The case was reopened and a new dental chart was prepared. During the process of preparing this chart, it was found that teeth had been charted incorrectly and dental work which had been done on the premolars had not been charted. Therefore, the case was now charted correctly. The police contacted the dentist of Linda Agostini, a Dr. O'Brien, who, when shown the correct chart and casts, positively identified the work done on her and an identification was made. However, to this day there is still no information as to who killed Linda, why she was burned, and how she turned up in the sack in the basement.

Similar situations can be avoided if the charting is done in a careful and meticulous manner.

Uses in Dental Identification

Dental records are of use in the identification by dentists of human remains in mass disasters and cases of mutilation of the human body beyond recognition by other means. In many of these cases, there is a clue as to who the victim may be, such as a passenger list of an airline. In some cases there may be no clues other than the teeth themselves.

In cases where there is a clue as to who the victim may be, the police should obtain from the possible family dentist the potential victim's chart along with any X-rays, models or other records. The department dentist will compare these with his own chart in an effort to obtain an identification. In the case where there is a list of possible victims, the name and address of the family dentist(s) of the victims should be obtained from their families. The dental chart of the possible victim from the family dentist should be obtained. The department's dentist will then compare the incoming charts with the charts he has made of the victims.

If the family dentist is unknown, but it is felt that the area or the region that the person is from is known, a copy of the chart should be sent to all dentists in the area for comparison with their charts. Hopefully, the dentists will check their own charts thoroughly and an identification will be made. If the number of dentists to whom the charts are sent is not too great, the police officer may follow up on the charts individually to see if the request has been given their attention. If this is impractical, as it would be in a large metropolitan area, a copy of the chart should be sent to the state and local dental societies in the city and state in which the dentist feels the person is most likely from. They will publish the chart in the local dental journal for the dentists to examine.

In some cases there are no clues as to the possible origin of the victim. In this case, a copy of the chart should be sent to the Journal of the American Dental Association in Chicago. The Journal will publish this chart. Hopefully, some dentist reading the Journal will see the chart, and it will remind him of one of his own patients, and he will check his charts and contact the department which placed the chart in the Journal. In all of these cases, a carefully prepared chart is obviously essential.

In cases where no specific identity is available for consideration, clues as to the region the person may be from can be such things as articles of jewelry, clothing, and the teeth themselves. The dentist can often tell what part of the country the person was from, or at least what the part of the country was in which the dentist of the victim was trained. The way in which he can do this is described below. If it is possible for the dentist to make this determination from the teeth, then it is possible to send the chart to the appropriate region's dental society for publication in their journal and also to send the chart to all dentists in the area where the body is found who were trained in that area of the country.

In some instances, it is also possible to obtain some clues as to the victim's possible occupation. The reason for that fact is that certain habits are common to certain occupations, such as chewing on pins among tailors, seamstresses, etc., and chewing on nails or holding nails in the mouth in the case of construction people. Over a period of years, this leaves characteristic notches or irregularities in the edge of the teeth. These, also, can be clues to the dentist(s) who receive the chart(s) as to the identity of the individual.

It is possible to gain some idea of where the person was from by the dental work because in spite of some similarities and a fair amount of overlapping, the type of dentistry practiced in one part of the United States varies to a greater or lesser degree from dentistry practiced elsewhere in the United States. East Coast dentistry differs from West Coast dentistry, which differs from Midwestern dentistry. American dentistry differs from Canadian dentistry, which is influenced by British techniques, and Swedish dentistry is quite different from Eastern European dentistry.

Silver fillings, in the case of the United States, on the East coast tend to be small, circular and as many as five or six may be placed on a single tooth. In the Midwest, silver fillings tend to be broad, perhaps extending across one-third the width of the tooth. Silver fillings in the Western United States are generally very narrow and very deep. Gold foil fillings, distinguished from inlays by their more yellowish color, are done more along the West coast than anywhere else in the country.

Partial gold crowns covering three-fourths of the area of the tooth (all but the front) are used instead of inlays in the Midwest and in the East. In California a type of crown covering seven-eighths of the tooth (all but a sliver of enamel on the front) is taught and occasionally constructed, but is rarely made anywhere else. Plastic veneer crowns (gold crowns with a white layer of plastic resembling the color of a normal tooth covering the gold on the front) are common throughout the South and Central Midwest, but the more expensive porcelain veneer crown (same but with porcelain instead of plastic for the facing) is more common in the East and in large metropolitan areas and in California. Solid gold crowns are generally placed on back teeth except among certain minority groups. Although rarely seen, some individuals have bizarre types of crowns, such as gold crowns with rhinestones set into them, or cutouts or gold inlays in various shapes, or with plastic facings in colors other than white. These unusual crowns can, in themselves, identify a person. Bridges are usually attached to crowns, but are occasionally constructed attached to inlays in the East, rarely in the Midwest, and never in the West.

Dentures provide less indication to the dentist of the region of origin than do fillings, crowns and bridges, but occasionally a denture or a partial denture will have the wearer's social security number or name either ground into an inconspicuous area on the denture or set into the plastic the denture is constructed from on a semitransparent plastic strip, which leads to an immediate and certain identification if found in the mouth. This practice should be actively encouraged among all dental laboratories and dental offices in the department's jurisdiction.

Whether the clues to identity were from a short list or whether the dentist had to evaluate the dental work to gain clues as to the regions of the country or the world to search for victim's identity, only half the job of dental identification is actually done by the dentist on the staff or retainer of the police department or the coroner's office and with their assistance. The other half of the work of dental identification is done by the dentist at work in the community, who must know his patients well enough and keep his records in such a way that he can easily refer to them and thus assist the authorities by finding charts and sending them in to the proper agencies for comparison and analysis. Without this cooperation from the average dentist in the community, few, if any dental identifications would ever be made. Fortunately, most dentists are quite eager to cooperate with the police whenever possible. It is obvious that the factor of chance could be partly eliminated by keeping microfilmed records of photographs of the dental arches along with the mugshots in some central location in each state or with the FBI, or more extensively, by computerizing the information. However, until this is done, clear and accurate charting will facilitate and enhance dental identification by the dentist, and the department will have done its part.

Chapter 5 __ __ __ __ __ __ __ __ __

PHOTOGRAPHS AND X-RAYS

— — — — — — — — — — — — —

PHOTOGRAPHS

PHOTOGRAPHY is one of the most important tools in law enforcement and is involved in many phases of the work of a police officer.

The process of photography was invented by a Frenchman named Daguerre in 1839 and was first applied to law enforcement by the Belgian gendarmes four years later, who started the practice of taking pictures of people they had arrested on criminal charges. These pictures were the first mugshots and were made on metal plates. Although they were primitive, they served their purpose well. This use of photography has survived to the present day.

Later, police began using photographs of the scenes of crimes and accidents, of bodies and wounds, and still later of documents and murder weapons. As the techniques of photography became more refined, police began taking photographs of the hair, paint chips, tire marks, tool marks and almost every kind of trace evidence imaginable. In this century, it has become possible to attach a camera to a microscope and take photographs of the microscope slide, which can be enlarged to show to an analyst or a jury.

Photography is also essential in the field of dental evidence in both the areas of dental identification and bite mark evidence. In the case of dental identification, the remains should be photographed on the site and at the morgue. Photographs of the dental arches may be used to supplement the dental charting to aid in confirming the identification. In the case of bite mark evidence, photography is especially important, as will be described in this chapter in detail.

When the police officer first interviews the victim of a sexual assault or any other violent crime, he should ask, among other things, whether the individual to his knowledge has been bitten. If the answer is in the affirmative, photographs should be taken, as will be described later in this chapter. It is conceivable that due to the location of some of the bite marks, the victim could be hesitant to display them to the police. Therefore, the person should be taken to a hospital and the doctor should be told either that bite marks are present, or if the victim's comments were inconclusive, the doctor should be asked to examine the individual for bite marks as a part of the general examination. Then, when bite marks are present, photographs should be taken in the presence of a doctor or a nurse. In this instance, both the police officer and the medical doctor should write down their own impressions in as concise and detailed a manner as possible. Photographs of bite marks should be taken, if possible, before the area which has been bitten is in any way bandaged, treated or manipulated except to the degree that is necessary to alleviate an emergency condition.

Since most medical doctors and pathologists prefer to refer to a dentist in dental matters, it is highly desirable that the police department should have a dentist on its staff who would be available to the department on very short notice to go either to the scene of a crime or to a hospital or to a morgue and supervise the part of the investigation relating to the dental evidence. When the dentist arrives, he should be told what photographs have already been taken, and he will indicate to the police photographer whether these will be adequate or whether he wishes additional photographs. It would be ideal for the dentist to be able to interview the victim firsthand in the hospital or to be taken to the scene if the victim is deceased, but the aforementioned photographs should be taken in any case in the event that the dentist is not able to arrive fast enough or on the chance that the department does not have a dentist available on short notice.

Types

The purpose of this section is to describe to the police photographer what types of photographs to take and when to take them. The general duty police officer should also be aware of the types of photographs which should be taken to preserve dental evidence. Since police photography is a well-established science in itself, it is beyond the scope of this book to describe the technical aspects of taking these photographs or to go into details of the equipment necessary. For those interested in reviewing the technical aspects of police photography several references are listed in the bibliography at the end of the book.

Police photography is nothing more nor less than good photography. A police photograph, in order to be valuable as evidence, must be absolutely stark and plain and honest. The important thing is that the photograph should exactly depict the scene at hand. It is generally not allowed to use special materials, lighting effects or lenses to hide or bring out certain details in a police photograph. In the area of dental evidence, where the photographs are being taken as an aid in identification, this rule should be followed. This is true also in the case of a bite mark, except that in this case it is necessary to arrange the lighting at various angles so that the indentations of the bite mark will be more definite on the photograph. It is also permissible to use filters to mask certain shades of color, mostly reds and blues associated with the bite mark, which might obscure the mark or blur the photograph.

British authorities have advised the use of a technique called stereoscopic photography to produce a picture which will show the details of the bite mark better. This is a very difficult procedure and involves an extensive amount of complicated equipment, and the results in most cases are not better than the results obtained in normal photography; therefore, the use of this technique is not advised.

It is important to remember that the bite mark should be photographed as soon as it is noticed. If a bite mark is found on a body at the scene, it should be photographed before the body is moved to the morgue. If the mark is discovered at autopsy, it should be photographed immediately, because human tissue degenerates rapidly with swelling, discoloration, destruction and breakdown of tissues which will mask and hide details of the mark and eventually obliterate it.

If the subject on whom the bite mark is found is alive, the body will attempt to repair the damage done by the bite mark. This process is called inflammation, and involves the production of heat, a red color and swelling, all of which can mask the bite mark and may make the photographic record less accurate. A bite mark on a live subject will remain clear and well-defined for from thirty minutes to thirty-six hours, depending on the amount of force with which the bite was inflicted, the part of the body on which the subject was bitten, and the type of tissue on which the bite was inflicted (whether there is muscle or bone underneath, whether there are large layers of fat underneath, or whether the victim has excess amounts of water in the tissues).

Types of Photographs

The three types of photographs used in dental evidence are black-and-white, color and infrared. The situations in which these types are best used are described below.

Black-and-White Photographs

Any good black-and-white film may be used for black-and-white photographs in the area of dental evidence. There are three considerations to bear in mind in the choice of a black-and-white film. First is the contrast, second the speed, and third the graininess.

CONTRAST. A film should be selected which shows a low degree of contrast and a broad, gray spectrum which, even though it is in black-and-white, will depict any differences in color much more readily than a high contrast film.

SPEED. A high speed film should be chosen since this gives a greater latitude to the lighting conditions necessary to produce an acceptable photograph.

GRAININESS. A film should be selected which is relatively non-grainy. Graininess refers to the size of the particles of silver on films and on the developing paper which produce the color. If the particles are large, any enlargements of the negative will have a speckled effect on the print, and there will be a resulting loss in detail. There may be some difficulty reconciling graininess with speed because generally the faster the film, the grainier the film.

In the area of dental evidence the graininess of the film is more critical than the speed, since the objects to be photographed will rarely be moving very rapidly. So, if it becomes necessary to choose between a fast film and one that has a very fine grain size, the film with the finer grain size should be selected. A film with smaller grain size will not only show more detail, but produces higher quality enlargements. This is important, because occasionally it will be necessary to have photographs enlarged to life size.

Color Photographs

There are three general types of color film: color-blind film, panchromatic film and orthochromatic film.

COLOR-BLIND FILM. Color-blind film registers only blue, violet and ultraviolet colors, and shows all other colors as black or white, and consequently is not useful in the area of dental evidence.

PANCHROMATIC FILM. Panchromatic film is sensitive to the entire range of colors. There are two types of panchromatic color films: type B, which registers colors in much the same way as the human eye does, and type C, which registers color in much the same way that the human eye does but is especially sensitive to yellows and reds. For recording dental evidence, a type C panchromatic film should be used.

ORTHOCHROMATIC FILM. Orthochromatic film does not register red light. Objects which are photographed on orthochromatic film and are red or tinted with red will appear black, whether filters are used or not. This type of film should not be used in the field of dental evidence for reasons which will be described later in this chapter.

Infrared Photographs

Waves of radiation on the longwave side of the visible light spectrum are called infrared rays. Infrared waves are unique because they are easily absorbed and changed into heat. Infrared waves are not heat rays, but they are associated with heat rays. Heat has nothing to do with light, but as heat is given off, the molecules of the object are made to vibrate faster on the surfaces and this gives off electromagnetic energy, and electromagnetic energy produces some infrared rays as long as the temperature of the object is above absolute zero. Since absolute zero exists only under laboratory conditions, everything gives off some infrared rays. The hotter an object's temperature is, the more infrared rays are given off. Although infrared rays are invisible to the human eye and are not colored red, they are visible to certain special types of film.

Infrared photography is useful in the field of dental evidence in situations when black-and-white or color film may be only of limited value. The situations in which infrared film should be used will be discussed later in this chapter.

Filters

A filter is simply a piece of colored glass which may be attached to the camera in front of the lens, which prevents any colored light of the same color of the lens from entering the camera. The most commonly used filters will be red or blue in this field of dental evidence for reasons described below.

Types of Cases

Before any photographs are taken, it is necessary for the officer present to describe in writing the scene to be photographed as he sees it. This should be done in all instances to lay the foundation for the use of photographs as evidence. There are no exceptions to this rule. Below are described the situations in the area of dental evidence when photographs are needed, with the types of photographs desirable.

Dental Identification

In the area of dental identifications, black-and-white photographs should be taken where the remains are discovered and at the morgue, as well as occasionally during the autopsy and the dental procedures involved in preparing a mouth chart, especially if access to the mouth involves surgical procedures on the part of the dentist or the pathologist, as is often the case with burn victims. Photographs should also be taken of the upper and lower dental arches, from straight above if possible, and from each side as an adjunct record to the dentist's chart. If it is impossible to take photographs from above the upper or lower dental arches, mirrors can be used to achieve the same effect. If the upper and lower jawbones and dental apparatus are physically removed by the doctors at the end of the autopsy procedure, photographs should be taken when the preparation of the bones has been completed of these from the front and from each side, and from directly above the upper and lower dental arches separately. If any casts are made from impressions of the dental apparatus, photographs should be taken of the models, together from the front and from each side, and separately from straight above.

Color and infrared films do not have to be used to record this type of evidence.

Bite Mark Evidence

BLACK-AND-WHITE PHOTOGRAPHS. No matter what other types of photographs are taken, black-and-white photographs should be taken in all instances. Other types of photographs should not be substituted for black-and-white photographs, but should be taken in addition to black-and-white photographs when indicated. When bite mark evidence is present, a piece of adhesive tape marked as a millimeter ruler should be placed below a bite mark in an area where it does not obscure the mark, so that it may be used as a reference guide in determining the actual size of the bite mark. Black-and-white photographs should be taken from directly above the mark and from every conceivable angle, and with as many different types of lighting as can be arranged to emphasize the outline and pattern of the mark, which may or may not be obscure. If there is a considerable amount of red or bluish-red discoloration and this discoloration serves not to delineate the position of the teeth, but tends to blur it, filtered black-and-white photographs may also be taken to mask the interfering color. If the predominant interfering color is red, a red filter should be used. If it is a bluish-black bruise, a blue filter should be used. It must be remembered, however, that when the bite mark is clearly delineated by red marks, filters should not be used.

COLOR PHOTOGRAPHS. In recording bite mark evidence, color photographs are desirable in addition to the black-and-white filtered and unfiltered photographs. These photographs should also be taken from directly above the bite mark and from every conceivable angle, and in as many different types of lighting as can be arranged to emphasize the bite mark.

Orthochromatic film, as described earlier, should never be used to record bite mark evidence for the following reasons: all bite marks are associated with a greater or lesser degree of reddish or reddish-bluish discoloration. Orthochromatic film is not sensitive to red colors, and any red or red-tinted object will show up as dark gray or black on orthochromatic film. Therefore, if there is any degree of reddish discoloration present and the photograph is taken using orthochromatic film, the entire area of the bite mark will appear dark gray to black and the film will be useless.

INFRARED PHOTOGRAPHS. Infrared photography is useful in recording bite mark evidence in the cases where the injury is so great as to produce enough discoloration and bruising from inflammation to mask a clear outline of the bite mark itself. The principle underlying infrared photography has already been described as being associated with the production of heat. When the body is damaged and inflammation occurs, heat is produced. The more severe the injury, the more heat produced. In the case of a large injury, the heat is often great enough to be felt, though it may not be associated with an increase in the person's temperature at first. The greatest amount of heat about an injury occurs where the greatest amount of inflammation is present. This is where the injury is greatest, which in the case of a bite mark is along the lines where the teeth produced their greatest force. Therefore, the increase in temperature is greatest at these points. Since the amount of inflammation and heat is greatest along the lines of the mark, the most infrared radiation will be produced there and will register on infrared film even though the area may be generally bruised.

Infrared photographs are very difficult to interpret and involve careful analysis because the picture can be complicated by nearby structures such as arteries and veins, but infrared photographs may often be the only photographic means of obtaining a usable record of a bite mark in the presence of severe general injury and discoloration.

Since infrared film is more expensive than standard color film, its use should be restricted to those instances when it is specifically requested by the consulting dentist. It should not be used in all cases, but in cases when it is indicated, it is indispensable. Therefore, the police photographer, as a precaution, should have with him a camera loaded with infrared film, should it be considered necessary by the dentist to use it.

The techniques of actually taking a photograph with infrared film may be found in any good book on photographic technique and are beyond the scope of this book.

All photographs, once taken, should be enlarged to life size and both the originals and the life-size enlargements should be made available to the dentist for analysis. The dentist will analyze the series of photographs and will determine which are useful and which are not, although none should be disposed of. The dentist will place sheets of acetate paper over the photographs and carefully trace the positions of the teeth on the photographs onto the transparent over-lay of acetate. He will then determine which marks represent which teeth, and these will be compared with the bite registration and models and casts obtained from the teeth.

Miscellaneous Physical Evidence

Items of physical evidence such as cheese or candy bearing tooth impressions, chewing gum bearing tooth impressions, or more rarely, items of food or other articles bearing portions of teeth in them, should be photographed in black-and-white from the angle and under appropriate lighting that best displays the impression of the teeth or the imbedded tooth. In the case of bite marks in food, as opposed to other physical evidence containing portions of teeth, color photographs should also be taken from the same angles and under the same conditions of lighting used for the black-and-white photographs.

Uses for Police

Photography is useful in the area of dental identification as a means of providing a visual record of the conditions of the mouth. They are an addition to, but not a replacement of, the chart com-piled by the dentist. During the procedure of compiling the dental chart and especially if any surgical procedures are done to gain access to the jaws at autopsy, photographs make a valuable perma-nent record of the procedure.

Photographs of the dental remains show more about the mouth than the chart can indicate and may be compared with the charts of dentists who may have treated the victim and thus be a valuable aid in making an identification. They may also be shown to a den-tist thought to have possibly treated the victim, since dentists often recognize their own work; in this way they may also aid in making an identification.

Photography is especially useful in the field of dental evidence in cases involving bite mark evidence such as battery, rape, homicide, or any combination of these; child abuse; or instances where the bite mark is in an item of physical evidence. This is because not everyone knows what a bite mark is or what it looks like. One per-son may think that a bite mark would look like a half-round row of marks on the skin, very clean and neat, another that it looks like a bruise. In real life, no matter how detailed the explanation of the bite marks with associated bruises and cuts, most people are unfamiliar with them. It will be found that the images people form when a bite mark is described verbally range from something resembling the actual bite mark to more often something quite different. A picture can greatly facilitate a full explanation of the type and nature of the bite mark and the injury, the damage and tissue destruction, and can demonstrate the alignment of the teeth, measure the spaces between the teeth, the width of the teeth, and can show the judge and jury the actual appearance the victim presented with.

As stated repeatedly, a picture does not eliminate the need for a detailed written description made by the officer present at the time when this picture is taken of the bite mark. Photographs, along with X-rays or models, which will be discussed later, may be admitted as evidence in court only as an addition to verbal or written testimony, because they are considered only to assist in the explanation. The person who took the picture, the dentist who evaluated it, and the officer present at the time the picture was taken, should be present to testify in court that the picture shown accurately portrays what it seems to show.

X-RAYS

X-rays are similar to light waves, except that they have a much shorter wave length than visible light. X-ray photography is based on the same basic principles as ordinary photography except that X-ray radiation is used instead of light waves to produce an image on film. X-ray photography requires special equipment usually found only in hospitals or dental offices. The equipment, which may be of various sizes and types, has a vacuum tube through which an electric current is passed, producing X-rays which cause a chemical change in a silver emulsion on film. Contrary to popular belief, X-rays will not pass through everything. An item which will permit X-rays to pass through is called "radiolucent"; an object which absorbs X-rays is called "radiopaque." Radiolucent objects appear on the X-ray as black areas. Radiopaque objects appear as white areas on an X-ray.

When an X-ray is taken, a film is placed behind the object to be photographed. The X-ray cone from which the X-rays emit is

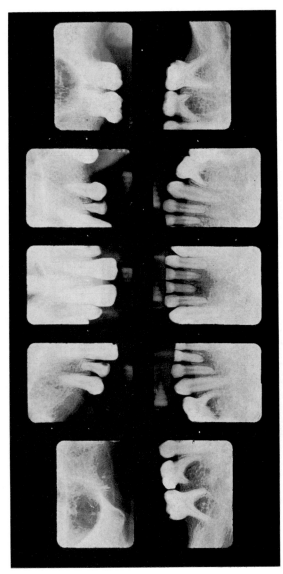

Figure 20. X-rays of a fourteen-year-old boy with complete hereditary absence of all but the upper front central permanent teeth. The absence of these teeth, the types and position of the roots present and the decay present can lead to an identification if compared with postmortem X-rays. (Courtesy of Edward Stafne: *Oral Roentgenographic Diagnosis*, 3rd ed. Philadelphia, Saunders, 1969, page 18.)

placed above the object to be photographed and the X-ray machine is turned on for a length of time. The length of time the machine is on determines the sharpness and clarity of the object photographed. Once the picture is taken, the X-ray film is developed in a way similar to that of ordinary film, although some different chemicals are used and a little different type of developer and fixing tank is used.

When analyzed by the dentist, the X-rays are developed to the negative stage. Positive prints are never used. The films are used as negatives with the objects that are dense and which absorb X-rays appearing as white objects, and objects which allow the X-rays to pass through as black objects. Objects in between will absorb varying amounts of X-rays and will appear in shades of gray.

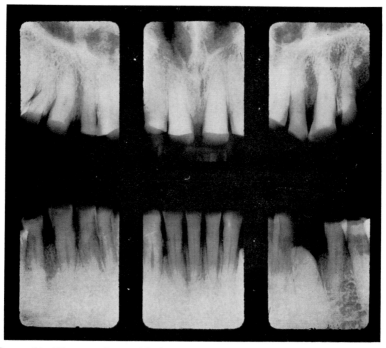

Figure 21. X-rays of an elderly person with considerable loss of tooth structure from abrasion and filling in of the pulp. This, plus the unusual tooth positions, can yield an identification if compared with postmortem X-rays. (Courtesy of Edward Stafne: *Oral Roentgenographic Diagnosis*, 3rd ed. Philadelphia, Saunders, 1969, page 61.)

The police officer should be aware of the fact that dental X-rays should be taken of the dental components of unidentified human remains. He should know what types of X-rays are needed so that in the absence of the dentist he can ask the medical examiner or coroner's pathologist to order the necessary films.

Police may not order X-rays to be taken; they can only be ordered on the prescription of a licensed dentist, M.D. or osteopath, although the officer may assist the trained medical or paradental personnel taking the films, if they so request. The actual techniques involved in taking X-rays requires long and exacting training and as such is limited to dentists and their specially trained assistants or medical X-ray technicians.

Only a dentist and no one else should read and interpret dental

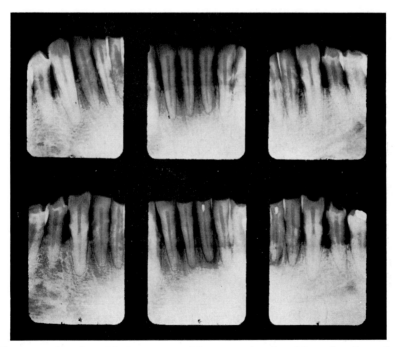

Figure 22. Another elderly person with severe abrasion. Note that the pulps have not filled in and that the tooth alignment is different, and bone is gone from around the ends of some teeth. Obviously this set of X-rays is from a different person than the X-rays in Figure 21. (Courtesy of Edward Stafne: *Oral Roentgenographic Diagnosis*, 3rd ed. Philadelphia, Saunders, 1969, page 61.)

X-rays. The police should see that the X-ray films, when taken, are properly mounted and taken to the dentist for evaluation.

Types

Different types of X-ray films are available which vary in the amount and contrast of black-and-white they will produce. The best films are those which have what is called the long gray scale: films that have a low contrast and allow much variation in the type of gray colors produced by the differing amounts of X-rays allowed to pass through. These films show much more detail and are easier to analyze, although to a casual observer they may appear less clear. As is the case with any photographs, X-ray films can be in or out of focus, which has nothing to do with the contrast between black-and-white of the film. Whether or not an X-ray film is in focus depends on how far the X-ray machine is from the film, the thickness of the object being X-rayed, the density of the object being X-rayed, and the amount of radiation emitted from the machine. All X-ray machines have controls to vary the amount of radiation produced; an incorrect setting will produce an X-ray that is out of focus.

Types of X-rays

There are basically four types of X-rays used in the field of dental evidence: head plates, panoramic X-rays, cephalometric X-rays and periapical X-rays.

Head Plates

A head plate is a large, flat photographic X-ray of the head. A lateral head plate is a flat X-ray showing a side view of one-half of the head. Both right and left head plates should be ordered, as well as a frontal head plate, which is a flat view of the front of the head. These X-rays are complicated to analyze, because there is some superimposition of structures on the opposite side of the head of each film.

Head plate films are used in the area of dental identification to provide a view of the interior structures of the teeth and jaws which can be compared with antemortem X-rays when obtained from a family dentist.

Panoramic X-rays

The panoramic X-ray is a long, narrow X-ray showing a cross

view of the middle one-third of the face, including the teeth and other dental structures. The panoramic film will show the area from approximately the upper part of the jaw joint and the lower rim of the eye sockets down to the lower border of the jaw, and an area from approximately the front of the right ear to the front of the left ear. Because the panoramic X-ray machine moves in the middle of the cycle to switch from the right side to the left side, or vice versa, there is always a blurred area in the center of the film. However, the machine is set up in such a way that the picture of the right side includes a portion of the left, and vice versa, so that by cutting the blurred portion out and moving the film together, one can obtain a complete, unobstructed view of the entire mid-facial area.

Panoramic X-rays are used to provide a complete panoramic view of the upper and lower jaws and all teeth and all associated structures. Panoramic X-rays are much easier to analyze than lateral head plates. A disadvantage of panoramic films is the fact that the upper and lower jawbones must be removed from the corpse at autopsy before this type of film may be taken, or the operator must be dealing with a skeleton.

Cephalometric X-rays

A cephalometric X-ray is a special type of lateral head plate taken on a special type of X-ray machine called a cephalostat. A cephalometric X-ray is always lined up on one specific landmark, usually the openings of the ears. All X-rays are superimposed on this point. If this type of rare X-ray is ordered by the medical pathologist or dentist, it will be necessary to obtain the services of a dental specialist in either orthodontics or pedodontics to analyze it, because the analysis of this film is complicated beyond the training of the general dentist.

Cephalometric X-rays are rarely used in the area of dental evidence because, due to the specialized equipment necessary to obtain cephalometric X-rays, the remains must be skeletonized. They are useful in the field of dental identification when the remains are those of a child or a teenager who, in the opinion of the dentist, may have had orthodontic or interceptive orthodontic treatment. The cephalometric X-ray obtained would be compared with existing cephalometric X-rays obtained from the family dentist, pedodontist or orthodontist.

Periapical X-rays

A periapical X-ray is simply a standard dental X-ray. The film is rectangular, measuring approximately one and one-half inches times three-fourths inch, and comes in two sizes, the aforementioned adult size, and a child size, which is slightly smaller. This type of X-ray may be taken using a film holder to position the film in the mouth of the subject, either in a standard dental office, or at the morgue using a portable miniature X-ray machine.

Periapical films may be taken in cases of dental identification in almost all instances where there are jaws, or teeth, or fragments of

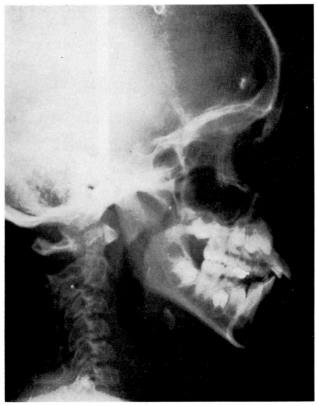

Figure 23. A typical cephalometric X-ray. (Courtesy of Ralph McDonald: *Dentistry for the Child and Adolescent*, St. Louis, Mosby, 1969, page 307.)

teeth present. A number of types of wooden or plastic X-ray holders, available from any dental supply house, can be used to position the film, whether the body is intact, partially decomposed, or skeletonized. The X-rays thus obtained are compared with periapical X-rays taken as a routine diagnostic service when these X-rays are obtained by the police from the family dentist. When only fragments of teeth or portions of teeth are recovered, as after a severe fire, these fragments may be placed on periapical films and individually X-rayed. The films thus obtained may then be compared with antemorten films obtained from the family dentist, and may in themselves effect an identification since they may show idiosyncrasies in root canal fillings or in the cavity preparations, or other idiosyncrasies of anatomy or of any fillings or crowns present such as overhangs or unusual carvings which may otherwise not be readily noticed.

Types of Cases

X-rays are generally used as an aid to the dentist in determining the identity of unidentified remains. They are not useful for interpreting bite mark evidence. When unidentified remains are found and taken to the morgue, mortuary or hospital, the dentist or medical pathologist will, in addition to other procedures, order either a panoramic X-ray or a set or right and left head plates. In the case of children or teenagers, he may order cephalometric X-rays or full lateral head plates.

When the police officer first contacts the dentist, at the time he is called into the case, after describing in detail the type, nature and quantity of the remains and the type of case, he should ask the dentist which X-rays he would like to have taken and transmit this information to the medical pathologist, so that the X-rays, if possible, may be taken while the dentist is on the way. The dentist may desire, when the remains are completely skeletonized, to have the remains brought to his office for examination rather than to the morgue. If the coroner is agreeable to this, the officer should bring the remains to the office, and the X-rays will be taken there on the dentist's own equipment at the time he prepares the chart.

In instances when the dentist may not be immediately reached, although the police officer may not under any circumstances order X-rays to be taken, he may inform the coroner/deputy coroner that the dentist usually wants X-rays to be taken so that there is a radiographic record of the entire dental structure and/or all teeth or tooth fragments and jaw fragments, and ask if he would like to order these X-rays or if he would prefer to wait until the dentist arrives to order the necessary films. In most cases, the coroner/deputy coroner will himself then order the films.

Situations occasionally arise, especially after mass disasters, in which the police officer will be confronted with a mass of fragmentary remains, tooth chips, portions of the roots and crowns of teeth, and disarticulated bone fragments. These bone and tooth fragments should be X-rayed on orders of the dentist or medical pathologist because the X-rays in the case of tooth roots will indicate the presence of root canal fillings which will remain intact, or in the case of portions of the crowns of the teeth, types of fillings which can be matched with the dental treatment records of the people known to be missing.

Uses for Police

The dentist will analyze the X-rays for the presence of root canal fillings, pulp treatments which may show up on the X-ray, any unusual fillings, tumors in the jaw, evidences of orthodontic movements or severe gum disease pockets, and other types of pathology, and in the case of lateral head plates or cephalometric films, for the presence of unusual patterns of growth in the underlying bone structures. All these will aid in the identification of the remains. Also, through a careful examination of X-rays, it is possible for the dentist to determine the age of the individual in question to within three to six months if it is a child under eighteen, and within five years if it is an individual over eighteen. Often it is through dental means alone that identifications can be made, as in the case of a badly decomposed or otherwise markedly changed body when the only remaining intact structures are the teeth and bones.

It is of great use to the police to know which X-rays will be taken and in which cases, namely in the cases of unidentified human remains, and to make the remains available to the dentist.

Chapter 6 __ __ __ __ __ __ __ __ __

IMPRESSION MATERIALS
AND TECHNIQUES

__ __ __ __ __ __ __ __ __ __ __ __

A N IMPRESSION is a negative imprint of an object in a more or less stable plastic material. An impression can be taken of any object, but in the field of dental evidence, the impression will be a negative imprint either of the teeth or of the biting edges and biting surfaces of teeth, or of parts of the body containing the marks or imprints of teeth and of individual items of physical evidence bearing imprints left by the teeth or containing tooth fragments.

Taking an impression is the first step in the creation of a permanent record of the object the impression is made from. No matter which material or technique is used, the impression should be made very carefully, so that a stable and accurate record of the object is created.

Impressions must be made of the dental structures in cases when identification of unclaimed human remains is to be made by means of dental records. The impressions, along with the chart compiled by the dentist and any X-rays ordered, will form a permanent record to which the dentist may refer as he works to evaluate incoming material in his effort to establish a definite identification.

When bite mark evidence on either a victim or a suspect is found, impressions must be made of the bite mark after the saliva wash and photographs have been made. When suspects are apprehended, impressions must be made of the teeth of the suspect, and special small impressions called bite registrations, in which the suspect bites a thin wafer of a special type of wax, must also be taken for comparison with the photographs and casts from the impressions taken on the victim at the time. If the mark is on the suspect, these procedures should be performed on the victim. Photographs alone are often not adequate to render by themselves an adequate identification.

Most states have very restrictive laws regulating who may or may not take impressions in the mouth, although as a general rule, impressions on areas *outside* the mouth for record purposes may be taken by anyone trained to handle and manipulate the materials properly. Taking impressions and bite registrations *inside* the mouth by individuals designated as dental assistants and working with and under the supervision of a licensed dentist is allowed by the Dental Practice Acts of many states if they are made for record purposes only and as long as no appliances, such as dentures, partial dentures, or bridges are to be made on the casts derived from the impressions. Other states stipulate that no one but a dentist may take impressions inside the mouth for any purpose. In states where auxiliaries may take impressions inside the mouth, any police officer or evidence technician may be trained in the techniques of taking impressions in the mouth, and assuming that the police department has on its staff a licensed dentist as a consultant, that officer trained to take oral impressions may be legally considered a dental assistant, working under his supervision. In the latter instance, any impressions taken in the mouth on suspects or at autopsy must be done by a licensed dentist. In these states, the police may take impressions of bite marks on portions of the body or on items of physical evidence, but must defer to the dentist when impressions in the mouth must be obtained. Therefore, the police department should have on its staff, in at least a consultant capacity, a licensed dentist to take impressions. Appendix IV lists the states and indicates which states allow assistants (officers in this case) to take impressions and which do not. To avoid any violations of the Dental Practice Act of the state in which the department is located, reference should be made to this table before any department's personnel are allowed to take impressions or bite registrations in anyone's mouth.

If a police department does not have the materials and the equipment to take impressions, a dentist should be called. Dentists have in their offices all the materials necessary for this type of work, and all dentists have working relationships with laboratories where the impressions may be taken to have casts made from them. In the long run, however, it will be more economical for police departments to obtain the equipment necessary to take impressions at the very least, and they should, if possible, obtain the equipment and materials necessary to prepare most types of casts, the construction of which will be described in the next chapter.

A single police officer or evidence technician should be designated and trained, where state law permits, in the techniques of taking both oral and non-oral impressions and in the techniques necessary to construct casts from these impressions. The police officer and/or evidence technician so appointed and trained should be legally designated as a dental assistant working under the supervision and direction of a dentist on the staff of the police department. The dentist should direct any officer or evidence technician involved in the taking, processing and pouring up of any impressions, casts, models or other related types of records, as well as perform their evaluation and interpretation. The training of any assistants or technicians should also be his responsibility. Impressions made with rubber base type impression material, impressions made of objects such as portions of the human body, or items of physical evidence which require the construction of a custom tray and special impressions techniques, must be prepared in rather unusual ways, and it will be necessary for the dentist to work very closely with the technician to produce the desired result.

The police department, through its staff dentist, should maintain a working relationship with any of the dental schools in the area so that more complex specialized equipment may be made available for such technical procedures as determining the age of an individual from tooth fragments by such procedures as X-ray defraction or analysis of trace minerals.

This chapter will discuss impression materials and techniques used in the field of dental evidence, and a section on each material will consist of a description of the basic physical and chemical properties of the material in general followed by the techniques and uses for police of the material.

Impression materials are simply the plastic or semiplastic materials used to make a negative imprint of an object. The basic types of materials used for all kinds of impressions, both dental and otherwise, are plaster of paris (not used in dental evidence), impression plaster which is a modified plaster of paris, nonreversible hydrocolloid impression material (alginate hydrocolloid), reversible hydrocolloid material (also not used in dental evidence), polysulfide rubber base impression material, and silicone rubber base impression material. The basic physical and chemical characteristics of the dental impression materials and the way in which they are used will be described below.

IMPRESSION PLASTER

Impression plaster is one of the oldest and most accurate impression materials in dentistry. Impression plaster is nothing more than plaster of paris to which chemicals have been added to increase its setting time and other materials, such as cornstarch, have been added so the plaster can be easily removed from the cast once it sets. Chemicals are also sometimes added to control the expansion of the impression plaster as it sets.

Plaster

Plaster of paris, from which impression plaster is made, is a product made from gypsum. Gypsum is a mineral which has been mined for several hundred years, and is used mostly as a construction material. In spite of the fact that it has been used for centuries, there is still much we do not know about it. Plaster is made by refining gypsum. This is done by grinding the gypsum into a fine powder and heating it to temperatures between 230°F and 260°F. When this is done, some of the water present inside the gypsum crystals is evaporated, and a chemical reaction occurs. The result of this reaction is a slightly different type of crystal, which lacks the water found in normal gypsum. Because approximately one-half of the water found in the gypsum crystal is gone, this is called a hemihydrate, a Latin term literally meaning, half of the water.

There are two different types of hemihydrates: alpha hemihydrates, or stones; and beta hemihydrates, or plaster of paris. These types vary primarily in the size and shape of the crystals present in the plaster powder. The alpha hemihydrate is a very strong material and is less subject to changes in its dimensions in the presence of temperature changes or water in the air or with variations in the amount of water used to mix it. The beta hemihydrate, or plaster of paris, has large and irregularly shaped crystals, as contrasted with the thin, needle-like crystals in the alpha hemihydrate. Beta hemihydrate plaster is weaker, less accurate, and less stable than alpha hemihydrates. Depending on the purpose for which the plaster is to be used, commercial plasters and stone contain, in addition to the hemihydrate crystals, materials to speed up or slow down the setting time, to control the expansion and to weaken or strengthen the set plaster, and coloring agents.

When plaster of either type hemihydrate is mixed with water, a complex chain of chemical reactions occurs, resulting in the re-forming of small crystals of the original gypsum within the suspension of the plaster, and as these crystals grow, they become intermeshed. This results in a single mass of plaster with a large amount

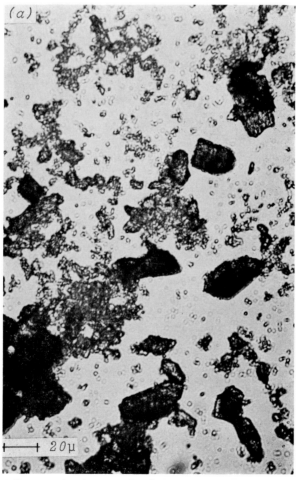

Figure 24. Microscopic photograph of three kinds of plaster particles. (a)

of water trapped in and between the crystals. This chemical reaction is complex, and its details are beyond the scope of this book.

Variables

The chemical setting reaction of plaster may be affected by several variable factors occurring during mixing: speed of mixing; ratio between the water and the powder used to mix the plaster; and temperature. The presence of certain additives during mixing or when manufactured is what makes plaster of paris into impres-

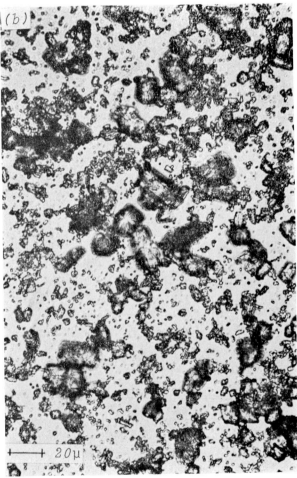

large coarse particles of plaster of paris (beta hemihydrate); (b) smaller, finer particles of dental stone (alpha hemihydrate); (c) crystals of gypsum

sion plaster. Additives may also be used to make the plaster useful for other purposes, such as cast plaster and die stone, discussed later. The presence of a chemical accelerator speeds up the setting time; the presence of a chemical retarder slows down the setting time. Even when the accelerators and retarders are added, the plaster is still vulnerable to the variables applying to ordinary plaster.

Mixing Time

The variations in the speed with which plaster is mixed affects

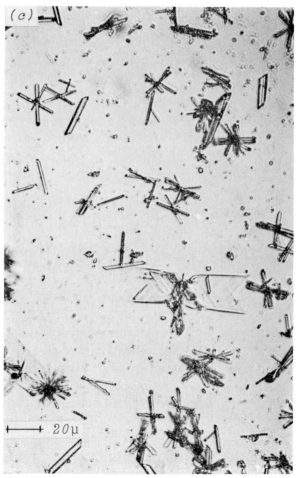

forming in a saturated solution of the material. (Courtesy of E. H. Greener, et al.: *Materials Science in Dentistry*, Baltimore, Wilkins, 1972, page 263.)

its setting time in the following way: the faster plaster is mixed the faster it sets. Given a constant amount of water and powder in the mix of plaster, assumed in this example to be a ratio of .45 as described below, if this standard mix of plaster is stirred for one minute before it is allowed to set, its setting time will be ten minutes. If it is stirred for three minutes, its setting time will be almost fifteen minutes, but if it is stirred for one-half minute, the plaster will set up in approximately five minutes.

The speed of mixing also affects the physical properties of the plaster once it has set in the following manner: The faster plaster is mixed and the faster it sets, the greater will be the amount of expansion and linear distortion and inaccuracies in the impression, if it is used as an impression material, and in the cast, if it is used as a cast material.

Water-Powder (W/P) Ratio

The water-powder ratio refers to the relationship expressed as a numerical ratio between the amount of water and powder used to mix plaster. The water-powder ratio affects the setting reaction of the plaster in a very simple way: the more water used, the longer it takes for the plaster to set.

The water-powder ratio is determined by dividing the weight in grams of water used to mix plaster by the weight of plaster powder the water is to be mixed with. This result is the water-powder ratio. For example, if 100 gms of plaster are mixed with 80 gms of water, the water-powder (W/P) ratio is .80; if 100 gms of plaster are mixed with 33 gms of water, the W/P ratio is .33; if 100 gms of plaster are mixed with 60 gms of water, the W/P ratio will be .60, and so forth. As an example of how the water-powder ratio affects the setting time of plaster, if a W/P ratio of .45 is used and a mixing time of one-half minute, the plaster will set in five minutes; if a W/P ratio of .80 is used and the mix is for one-half minute, the plaster will take approximately ten minutes to set.

The water-powder ratio also affects other physical properties in plaster besides the time necessary for the setting reaction to take place. The higher the water-powder ratio used, the less expansion that will occur in the plaster, but the plaster will be more porous and weaker and will exhibit less crushing strength. A lower water-powder ratio will produce more expansion, but will result in a denser and stronger mixture when the mixture has set.

Combinations of variations in water-powder ratio and setting time can be used to vary the setting time for individual purposes. For example, if a W/P ratio of .45 is used and a mixing time of one-half minute, the plaster will set in five minutes; if a W/P ratio of .80 is used and a mix for one minute, the setting time will be seven and one-half minutes; if a W/P ratio of .70 is used and the mix is for two minutes, setting time will be six minutes; if a W/P ratio of .40 is used and the mix is for one minute, the plaster will set in three minutes. In instances when it is desired that the plaster set up in a longer or shorter period of time or when more accuracy is required with less linear distortion and no specific type of plaster to which chemicals have been added to produce this effect is in supply, the judicious variation of water-powder ratio and mixing time can produce the desired effect.

Temperature

At room temperature there is little effect on the setting time of plaster. When the temperature of the mixture increases above 120°F, a slowdown of the set occurs. At temperatures of 194° to 212°F plaster will not set, but mixing of plaster at those temperatures is unlikely, so it need not be considered. As the temperature goes down, the plaster will set more and more slowly until the freezing point is reached. Changes in temperature have little effect on the final physical properties of the plaster, except those effects caused by a shorter or longer setting time, as described earlier. In order to vary the setting time, one may vary the temperature of the water the plaster will be mixed with. If a longer setting time is desired, cold water should be used. If a shorter setting time is desired, warm water should be used within limits. If the water is so hot as to make it uncomfortable to touch it should not be used for mixing plaster.

Accelerators

The most reliable means of controlling the setting time of plaster is with accelerators. An accelerator is a chemical added to the plaster powder which will increase the setting time. Potassium sulfate is the most commonly used accelerator. Many other chemical salts also act as accelerators, and on an ordinary, practical basis, table salt used in the concentration of one tablespoon per pint of water used to mix plaster will result in an acceleration of the setting time. However, in larger amounts, table salt can also act as a retarder.

The accelerators also have a considerable effect on the setting expansion. Chemicals such as potassium sulfate, sodium sulfate, alum, and terra alba have a strong effect on setting expansion, causing a great linear expansion. Terra alba is the worst material in this respect. Plasters made with terra alba as an accelerator should be avoided for forensic purposes.

Retarders

A retarder is a chemical added to plaster powder which has the function of slowing down the setting time. Commonly used retarders are borax and sodium citrate. Retarders are generally used in plasters in the building trades where setting time of thirty minutes to an hour and upwards is needed, but these have little application in dental evidence work. From the standpoint of dentistry, the setting time should be controlled very accurately. In forensics it is of more importance to control the setting expansion.

Setting Expansion

The setting expansion is defined as the amount of increase in linear dimensions that a mass of plaster undergoes as it changes from a liquid to a solid state. Most plasters undergo a linear expansion of from .06 percent to 5 percent. The expansion found in plaster of paris is on the high end of this scale; the amount of expansion found in dental stones, or alpha hemihydrates, is on the lower end of this scale. Most modern impression plasters exhibit a setting expansion of in the range from .04 percent to .07 percent.

Impression Plaster

A desirable impression plaster should exhibit the following properties: It should have a setting time in the range of from three to five minutes, depending on the water-powder ratio used; its setting expansion should be in the range of .04 percent to .07 percent. It should have the proper amount of accelerators and retarders added to the plaster powder itself, not in a separate jar accompanying the plaster of paris. Having to measure the proper amount of chemical modifiers and add them to the plaster in the case of impression plaster lengthens the procedure of mixing the plaster and adds an additional source of error, i.e. the possibility of variations in the amounts of chemical modifiers added to the plaster powder. Impression plaster should contain a material such as cornstarch or potato starch to render it more soluble when it is to be removed from the cast material. It should contain color pigments to differentiate the impression from the cast material as it is removed after the cast material has set.

A high water-powder ratio should be used with impression plaster to aid in the prevention of the formation of exothermic heat (heat given off by the chemical setting reaction of plaster). Because of the presence in the powder of chemical modifiers, this should not unduly affect the setting time. Exothermic heat could have an adverse effect on certain materials of which an impression is desired; it could damage or blister a portion of the body of which an impression is being made producing swelling, discoloration and inflammation which could obscure the bite marks present and render useless any infrared photographs taken of this area afterwards.

Dimensional Stability

Dental impression plaster is a reasonably stable material, although when it sets two things occur: first, although there is a decrease in volume on setting of 7 percent to 8 percent, there is actually a linear expansion of from 0.15 percent to 0.3 percent. This linear expansion is caused by the outward growth of the crystals of gypsum as they form in the plaster. The amount of setting expansion can be altered to a small degree on either the long or the short side by varying the water-powder ratio.

Availability and Storage

Impression plaster can be purchased from any dental supply house. It is usually available in either cans or drums containing from one to fifty pounds. Since this material has rather limited use as other more accurate and workable materials are currently available, only a small amount need be kept on hand by the department.

The only precaution which needs to be taken with the storage of the impression plaster is that the container should be kept tightly closed. Plaster will absorb moisture from the air over a period of time, and this will institute a very slow setting reaction and can destroy the properties of the material.

Techniques

The items of equipment necessary for the use of impression plaster impressions are:

1. a flexible rubber, round-bottomed mixing bowl;
2. a broad, flatbladed spatula with rounded ends (not square corners as they will not reach into all areas of the mixing bowl);
3. a mechanical vibrator, which is a rubber platform mounted on a small electronic motor;
4. a tray to carry the plaster, as described in Chapter 8. If the impression is to be taken in the mouth, a stock metal unperforated tray should be selected; if the impression is to be of another portion of the body or a piece of physical evidence, a custom tray should be constructed.

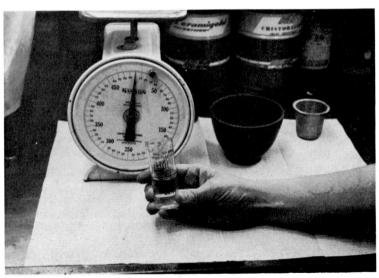

Figure 25. Water measure containing the right amount of water to give the correct water-powder ratio for mixing impression plaster.

Impression plaster should be mixed and utilized in the following manner:

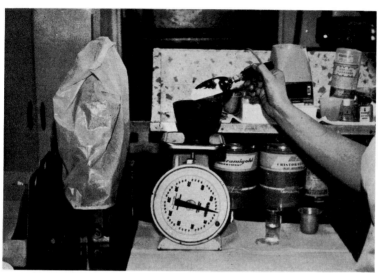

Figure 26. The proper amount of plaster is weighed to provide the correct amount to obtain the desired water-powder ratio. The powder will then be added to the water already measured.

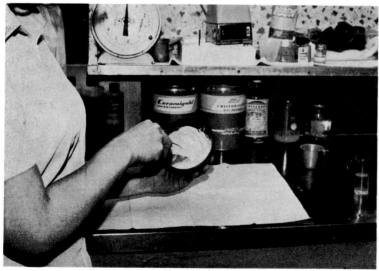

Figure 27. Impression plaster being mixed.

1. The proper amount of water should be measured according to the desired water-powder ratio.

2. The proper amount of plaster powder should be measured by weight in accordance with the desired water-powder ratio.

3. The plaster powder should be very slowly added to the water in the flexible mixing bowl.

4. With the rounded spatula, the mixture should be stirred vigorously until it is of a smooth, homogeneous consistency. The plaster should be mixed for at least one minute and for not more than three minutes. Remember that any increase in the mixing time will result in changes in the setting time and dimensional accuracy. As the plaster is mixed, it should not be merely stirred, but the edge of the spatula should be used to press the mass of plaster against the side of the mixing bowl with broad, sweeping motions while the mixing bowl is itself rotated slowly.

5. When the plaster is in a smooth, homogeneous state, it is placed on the mechanical vibrator. When the machine is turned on, the platform holding the bowl vibrates very rapidly causing any air incorporated in the mix to rise to

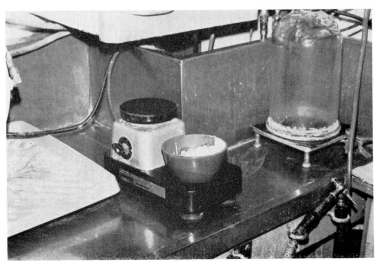

Figure 28. Bubbles in the plaster mix being vibrated to the surface and eliminated.

the surface. This will help prevent the inadvertent incorporation of bubbles into the plaster mix, which could result in voids in critical areas in the impression.

6. The stock or custom tray selected to carry the plaster impression material to the object of which the impression is to be taken should not be coated with an adhesive, because there are undercuts around the teeth in the mouth and in order to remove the set plaster it will be necessary to fracture the impression material in two or three key places and then reassemble it carefully and tightly in the tray, which would be impossible if the tray is coated with adhesive.

7. Small amounts of the impression plaster should be taken on the end of a spatula and gently vibrated into the tray. This is repeated again and again until the tray is filled. The tray, after each increment of plaster is added, should also be vibrated slightly to express any bubbles which may inadvertently have been entered into the mix. When the tray is filled, additional plaster should be added so that the tray is slightly overfilled with material.

8. The tray containing the impression plaster should be placed either in the mouth or over the object the impression is to

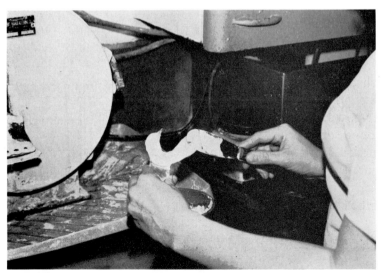

Figure 29. An impression tray being loaded with plaster.

be made of. It is placed on the object or against the teeth, seated very gently using firm pressure and a very slight amount of vibration. Once the tray is firmly in place, it should be held gently but firmly until the plaster sets, which may be determined when the plaster is no longer warm, or when it is no longer crumbly when scraped with a sharp instrument.

9. The tray is very gently removed. The mass of set impression plaster should come with the tray unless there are undercuts present on the object of which the impression was taken. If this is the case, the plaster should be scored with a sharp knife; either a laboratory knife or a large pocket knife may be used for this purpose. Then, with the edge of the knife on the plaster, it should be very gently tapped to cause a fracture and it should be removed from the object in sections to be reassembled in the tray.

10. After reassembly in the tray, a cast may be poured up on written orders of a dentist. The techniques for pouring a cast from this type of impression will be described in Chapter 7.

Uses for Police

Plaster of paris is traditionally used in law enforcement for such things as impressions of tire prints and footprints. However, plaster of paris is not acceptable for use with dental evidence due to its long setting time, the high amount of heat produced as it sets, and its dimensional instability. Impression plaster, while a good material which can be used in the field of dental evidence, has some disadvantages. Primary among these is the exact regulation of the water-powder ratio necessary since this material is not supplied in premeasured packets. Furthermore, if the object of which the impression is taken contains undercuts, impression plaster must be fractured and reassembled; this is a tedious, exacting job, requires considerable skill and time, and is an additional procedure that must be performed. While it is an inexpensive material, there are better and more convenient impression materials available today.

NONREVERSIBLE HYDROCOLLOID (ALGINATE) IMPRESSION MATERIAL

Before World War II, one of the most commonly used impression materials in dentistry, and a material incidentally totally unsuitable for forensic purposes, was one made from agar, which is a product made from kelp seaweed. During World War II, the importing of agar from Japan was stopped. Since there were no domestic sources of agar at that time, the residual supply became depleted, and what small amounts of this material were left were allocated entirely to medicine to make a culture medium for bacteriological studies. At that time, nonreversible hydrocolloid impression material, also called alginate, was developed as a substitute. and this material is used today as probably the most common general use impression material in dentistry. Its use today far exceeds that of any other impression material, and this material does have a use with dental evidence.

The main ingredient in nonreversible hydrocolloid impression material (alginate) is a member of the family of ingredients called alginate. It is a salt of alginic acid, which is a deritivite of kelp. It is a type of chemical chain called a polymer and has a complex chemical formula.

Alginic acid is not soluble in water, but some of its salts are, including some used for impression material. While most of the inorganic salts of alginic acid are not soluble in water, the salts obtained from sodium, potassium, ammonium, and magnesium alginic acids are soluble, and both sodium and potassium alginate are used extensively as impression material. This solubility has an important effect on its use.

Alginate impression material contains chemical accelerators or retarders. These chemicals are always an intrinsic part of the material. Alginate impression materials contain small amounts of calcium sulfate, which is a catalyst and intended to accelerate the setting reaction. Some alginates contain in addition to calcium sulfate, small amounts of sodium or potassium phosphate, oxylate or carbonate. Small amounts of these salts are used as retarders to give a finer control over the setting reaction.

Another material included in alginate impression material is a filler. This is added in precise amounts to increase the strength and stiffness of the material, to produce a smooth texture, and to insure a firm surface which is not sticky. Without the filler, which is generally diatomaceous earth, the gel is weak, flabby and sticky, with drops of water forming on the surface, and is totally unacceptable as an impression material.

All companies which make alginate impression materials have their own formulas, and these formulas are tightly kept industrial secrets. A typical alginate impression material, however, might consist of 10 percent potassium alginate, 79 percent diatomaceous earth, 10 percent calcium sulfate, and 1 percent trisodium phosphate as a retarder.

One difficulty with alginate impression material is that when plaster is poured against it to form a cast, the cast may have a soft surface as a result because the setting reaction of the plaster is retarded by its contact with the hydrocolloid. Therefore, chemicals such as sodium silicofluoride or potassium silicofluoride are added in small amounts to the above formulas to counter this effect and produce a better stone surface.

Variables

The physical properties of alginate impression material are affected by the mixing time, the water-powder ratio, and the temperature at which it is mixed and stored. The humidity of the immediate environment affects the dimensional stability of the set impression.

Mixing Time

The manufacturer's instructions should be followed closely regarding the length of time a particular brand of alginate hydrocolloid should be mixed. The strength of the final gel is reduced by as much as 50 percent if the mixing time is shorter than indicated. If it is not adequately mixed, there will be a failure of the ingredients to dissolve thoroughly, and the chemical reactions will not proceed at the same rate throughout the mass of material, causing some parts of the material to set earlier than others and resulting in distortions. If the alginate is mixed too long, some of the calcium alginate particles formed as the setting proceeds will be broken up and the strength of the material will be lowered, and the result will be a weak impression which could pull apart when it is removed. Alginate impression material should be mixed the exact length of time directed by the manufacturer and the mixing time should be checked with a watch if possible.

Water-Powder (W/P) Ratio

It is important with alginates to use the proper water-powder ratio as specified by the manufacturer. If too much water is used, the impression material will take an unusually long time to set, be very runny and weak, and when it is removed from the object will show a rapid shrinkage. If an inadequate amount of water is used, portions of the mix of alginate will remain in a powder form, unset, and other areas will imbibe the water and congeal. The result is a mass of useless material. This process can occur in a matter of seconds and make it necessary to prepare an entirely new mix of material.

Temperature

The effect of temperature on the setting reaction of alginate hydrocolloid impression material is dramatic during both mixing and storage of materials.

Water temperature has a great effect on the setting time of alginate; the higher the temperature, the shorter the setting time. For example, at boiling the setting time of an average alginate is one and one-half minutes. At body temperature of 98.6°F it is three minutes. At 77°F it is four minutes, and at 68°F it is four and one-half minutes, and at 63°F it is eight minutes.

The temperature also affects the viscosity and flow of the impression material. The higher the temperature, the shorter the period of time the material has a flow adequate for use as an impression material. The lower the temperature, the longer the period of time the material has an adequate flow for use as an impression material.

Some alginate impression materials are more sensitive to temperature change than others. Fast-setting alginates are much more affected by changes in temperature than is a slower setting gel. There are fast-setting alginates available which have as much as a twenty-second change in setting time for every degree of Centigrade change in temperature. In such cases the temperature of the mixing water must be regulated very carefully to within 1° to 2°C of a standard temperature. This type of material is so sensitive that it is impractical for police use because the likelihood of controlling the temperature of the mixing water so accurately is not high. A slower setting alginate impression material will be less affected by temperature than a fast-setting material, although it is well to remember that all alginates as a class of compounds are sensitive to temperature, and extremes of hot and cold should be avoided in the mixing water.

Alginates are affected by both the temperature of the mixing water and by the temperature of the environment in which they are mixed. Alginate materials mixed out-of-doors on a cold day (30°F or lower) will take much longer to set than alginates mixed out-of-doors on a hot summer day with a temperature of 110°F. Allowances should be made for these extremes of environmental temperature by using water temperatures to compensate. On a very hot day, use cool water; on a very cold day, use warm to hot water if the material is to be used outside of the mouth. If the material is to be used inside the mouth and mixed outdoors, the temperature of the water still may be varied from lukewarm to cool, but the variation should be less extreme because the body heat of the subject when the material is in the mouth will accelerate the set.

The physical properties of alginates after they are mixed are also affected by the temperature at which the powder is stored. When alginate impression material has been stored for as little as thirty days at a temperature of 90°F on the average, the material is unsuitable for use. It will either fail to set up at all or will set up much too rapidly. If it is stored at 80°F for a month, there will be evidence of deterioration in the form of a very rapid set or a retarded set, but the material will be usable, although only barely so. Alginate impression material should be stored at cool temperatures in the range of 50° to 70°F and never kept for any prolonged period at any temperature above 75°F.

Dimensional Stability

The dimensional stability of alginate hydrocolloid impression material is notoriously poor. After an alginate impression is removed from either the mouth or the object of which the impression is taken, although the material is set sufficiently for removal and cast construction, the chemical reaction of setting continues for some time, producing an expansion of approximately .1 percent during the first half hour. Then the material begins to shrink, even if the impression is kept in an atmosphere of 100 percent humidity. Under such conditions, after one hour the material will have recovered from its original expansion and will be the same size it was when it was removed from the object of which the impression was taken. However, after two hours, the material will have shrunk by .3 percent and the shrinkage will continue slowly. When the material is exposed to the air, the shrinkage will continue at a much faster rate, until at the end of twelve to thirty-six hours, depending on the temperature, the material may have shrunk by 25 to 30 percent. After a week, the shrinkage may be as high as 50 to 60 percent. In addition to conditions of storage, improper water-powder ratio may cause rapid shrinkage upon removal of the impression from the object.

It is of utmost importance that care be taken in the manipulation of this material to minimize the dimensional instability. For example, an impression of a bite mark could be taken on a person or an object and improper manipulation of the material could result in a cast of the bite either much larger or much smaller than it actually was. The person who actually perpetrated the crime and left the bite mark might then be apprehended, and an accurate impression of his mouth would not quite fit the impression obtained at the scene. Chances are the suspect would have some irregularity of alignment, distinctive spaces, or unusual tooth positions, and in all probability an identification could at least tentatively be determined, but the fact that the bite registration and the casts of the suspect did not quite fit the bite marks or quite match with the bite mark impressions would provide the defense attorney an opportunity to attempt to impeach the evidence or to place doubt concerning this type of evidence in the minds of the jurors. This problem can be greatly decreased by careful manipulation of the materials.

Availability and Storage

Alginate impression material can be purchased by a police department either in individually sealed packets, each packet containing a sufficient amount of preweighed powder for an individual impression, or it may be purchased in bulk form in a can. Although the material is less expensive in bulk form, it is difficult with this to prevent variations in the water-powder ratio. The individual premeasured packets are better because there is less chance of contamination during storage and the exact water-powder ratio is assured. Plastic cups are provided by the manufacturer for the proper measurement of the water. This system is foolproof.

Alginate impression materials should always be stored at cool temperatures in the range of 50° to 70°F. They should never be kept for any prolonged period of time at any temperature above 75°F. The reasons for this are discussed under Temperature.

Techniques

The following materials are needed for the preparation of an alginate impression:

1. a flexible, rounded rubber mixing bowl of a size to fit comfortably in the hands;
2. a broad, flatbladed spatula with rounded ends;
3. a tray to carry the alginate to the object of the impression, selected (and constructed if it is a custom tray) as described in Chapter 8, and
4. a premeasured packet of alginate in the amount desired.

When mixing alginate impression material, it is important to remember that there are differences in manipulation made necessary by the differences in setting time and working time between different proprietary brands of alginate, so it is important to check with the manufacturer's brochure and follow the manufacturer's instructions. However, in general alginate impression material is prepared for use and utilized in the following manner:

1. The proper amount of water to mix the stated amount of alginate in the correct water-powder ratio should be measured and poured into the rubber bowl.
2. The properly measured amount of alginate should be added slowly to this water.
3. The mixture should be vigorously stirred. The length of time the alginate is to be stirred is dependent on the brand and the characteristics of the particular type of alginate used. However, after a thorough mixing the alginate should be very smooth and without any graininess. The smoothness of the material will vary considerably from one manufacturer to

another, so it will be necessary to experiment with the brand
of alginate purchased to become thoroughly acquainted with

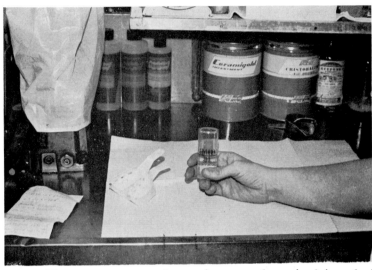

Figure 30. The proper amount of water is measured to mix alginate hydro-colloid impression material.

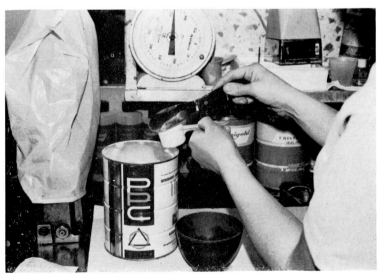

Figure 31. The proper amount of alginate powder is measured with a special scoop supplied by the manufacturer. It should be filled even with the top, but not beyond.

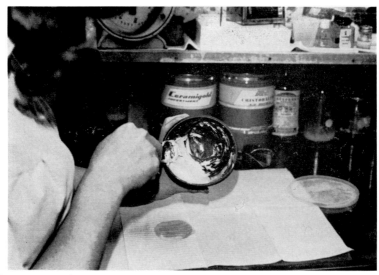

Figure 32. Alginate hydrocolloid being mixed with a rounded spatula in a flexible rubber bowl.

its properties. Generally a smooth, creamy texture will be obtained with any of the better commercial products.

4. The properly mixed alginate should be taken in small amounts on the end of the blade of the spatula and carried to the tray

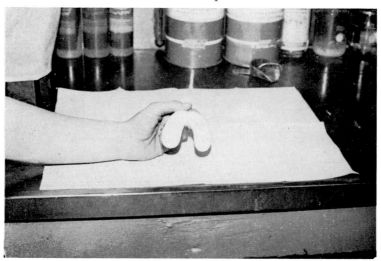

Figure 33. An impression tray filled with alginate hydrocolloid impression material.

and placed into the tray with a slight amount of pressure to express some of the alginate material through the perforations of the tray. More alginate is carried to the tray until the tray is slightly overfilled.

5. The tray should be carried to the mouth or the object of which the impression is to be taken and gently but firmly seated. The impression must be held in place with light pressure until the material has set. The material has set when it no longer feels soft to the touch, but feels firm and resilient.

6. When the alginate is set, it should be removed from either the mouth or from the object of which the impression is taken using a quick snap. The material should not be removed using a slow, steady pull because this will result in more distortion than a quick tug or snap. It is important that the tray not be

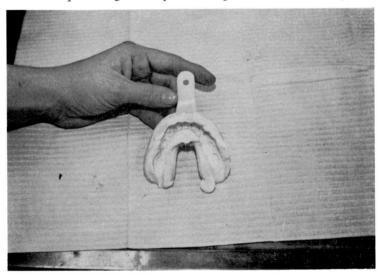

Figure 34. A completed alginate hydrocolloid impression.

removed from the impression object too early, before the set is complete; this will produce a roughened, pitted surface in the cast. On the other hand, the alginate material should not be held in place too long either; there are alginate materials on the market which, if held against the impression object for five minutes longer than they are supposed to be held will distort significantly.

7. The alginate impression should be poured up with cast material within one-half hour at the longest, but preferably within fifteen minutes, and no sooner than five minutes after removal.

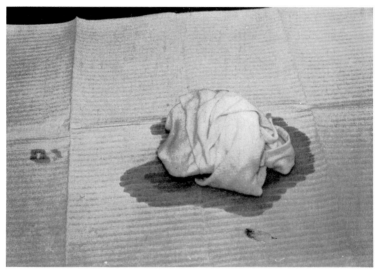

Figure 35. An alginate impression should be wrapped in a wet towel until it is poured up with plaster or stone.

In the interim period between its removal from the object or person and the time it is poured up, it should be kept moist with a moist paper towel or napkin to provide an atmosphere of 100 percent humidity. It should not, however, be immersed in water. Under the wet paper towel the water lost into the air by the alginate will be replaced by the water in the towel, but immersed in water the alginate has only the opportunity to soak up water, not also to lose water into the air, so the impression would most likely expand.

These measures will assure that this dimensionally unstable material will be optimally accurate. Any deviations from this important last procedure will severely compromise the usefulness of the impression.

Uses for Police

Alginate impression material is a very useful and versatile material and should be included among the supplies of every police department laboratory. It is very easy to use once the technique has been learned, easily stored if the temperature is kept under control, and much less messy than some of the more accurate impression materials to be described later. Alginate impression material is relatively inexpensive.

Although when handled poorly alginate will distort badly, it is a very accurate material when properly used. An alginate which meets the American Dental Association's current specifications will reproduce a line .0015 inches in width, which is more accurate than plaster impression material but less accurate than rubber and silicone base impression materials. Alginate is a very versatile and accurate impression material for primary casts for record purposes and for primary casts obtained for analysis by the dentist. In many cases, a more accurate impression is desired, particularly of the mouth and of certain types of perishable physical evidence, and for these a more accurate material such as the rubber base material or silicone material is used. However, alginate may be used to prepare impressions for casts on which customized trays of acrylic may be constructed as described in Chapter 8 to carry some of the still more accurate materials.

RUBBER BASE IMPRESSION MATERIALS
POLYSULFIDE RUBBER BASE IMPRESSION MATERIAL

Commonly known simply as rubber base impression material, this type of preparation is made of synthetic rubber, usually a mercapton or polysulfide rubber, which sets into a mass of artificial rubber suitable for use as an impression material by reaction with a catalyst. Polysulfide rubber impression material has been developed for the most part since World War II and it is closely related to many other types of polysulfide rubber which have found wide application in industry.

Most polysulfide rubbers consist of a rubber base paste and an accelerator paste which are both made of a number of components. Of primary importance in the base paste is a polysulfide polymer (or long chain of rubber molecules) in the form of a liquid. Zinc oxide and calcium sulfate powders are added to the polymer to make it into a workable paste. The zinc oxide and calcium sulfide are referred to as fillers or extenders when combined with rubber base material because they are completely inert and do not in any way enter into the vulcanizing reaction, also known as the setting or curing reaction.

Most rubber base pastes also contain very small amounts of silica. The silica is ground into a very small particle size. It is used as a reinforcing agent and it is thought to enter into the crystal structure itself to reinforce the rubber and make it more elastic. The silica is sometimes included in the accelerator instead of the base paste.

As with alginates, intrinsic to the composition of the rubber material is the accelerator, in this case in the form of a paste which is combined with the base to produce the ready-for-use material. The accelerator paste usually contains lead peroxide as a catalyst, small amounts of sulphur and castor oil. The lead peroxide catalyst is necessary to initiate the setting or vulcanizing reaction. When it is mixed with the rubber base material a long and complicated chain of chemical reactions occur during which there is a slight rise in the temperature of the mix and varying amounts of hydrogen gas is given off. While the catalyst does contain lead, it is not toxic, at least during the time the material is in the mouth. A small amount of sulphur included in the accelerator paste is intended to provide a more workable material with more stable physical properties.

Both lead peroxide and sulphur are powders. Due to the consistency of the base paste and the amount of accelerator needed, it is necessary that the accelerator compound also be a paste. Therefore, some material must be added to these powders to turn the mixture into paste, and this material is usually castor oil. Some commercial products also include small amounts of stearic acid to control the vulcanizing time and mask the unpleasant hydrogen sulfide odor produced as the setting reaction progresses, and chromium oxide or a similar chemical as a hydrogen acceptor to attract and bind the extra hydrogen gas produced by the chemical reaction forming the rubber. The resultant compound of chromium oxide and hydrogen becomes a part of the rubber material itself and does not in any important way affect the final physical properties of this material.

Variables

The physical properties of polysulfide rubber impression material are affected by a number of factors: mixing time, the ratio of base to accelerator, temperature and humidity.

Mixing Time

Unlike plasters and nonreversible alginate hydrocolloid, rubber base impression material is not greatly affected by variations in the mixing time. If the material is mixed too long, it will simply set up on the pad and the spatula will be stuck in it. If the material is mixed for an inadequate period of time, a complete mixing of the materials will not be achieved and there will be pockets of unmixed and unreacted base and accelerator throughout the mix with resulting weak spots, voids and rough areas throughout the impression, but the setting time will be the same.

Base-Accelerator Ratio

Just as plaster and nonreversible alginate hydrocolloid are considerably affected by changes in the water-powder ratio, in a similar fashion rubber base material is greatly affected by variations in the ratio between base material and accelerator material. Because the chance for error in mixing the proper proportions of the material is so great, this material is prepared by the manufacturer in tubes with openings regulated and gauged so that when equal lengths of material are squeezed from a tube on a pad they will be in the proper proportions for an ideal mix.

The working time and setting time of polysulfide rubber base impression material can be controlled to a certain extent by varying the length of the accelerator material in proportion to the base material by as much as one-third either way on the long or the short side. If the length of accelerator material equals one and one-third the length of the rubber base material, the set will occur faster. If the accelerator is varied by one-third less than the equal amount to the base, the material will set up slower. If the amount of accelerator is varied to a greater extent than this, however, the mechanical properties of the material will be destroyed and the result will be either a rubber which sets up too fast, is too stiff and thus unworkable, or a rubber which is not stiff enough, resulting in gross inaccuracies in the casts poured up from these impressions.

Setting Time

The working time and setting time of polysulfide rubber impression material, as is the case of plaster and alginate, varies somewhat from manufacturer to manufacturer since the exact ingredients and proportions of ingredients in the different parts vary from manufacturer to manufacturer. The working time of a polysulfide rubber impression can be from three minutes to ten minutes and its setting time from four and one-half minutes to twelve minutes. On an average the working time of a rubber base impression material at a room temperature of 78°F can be expected to be nine minutes and the average setting time at mouth temperature of 98.6°F can be expected to be about five minutes.

Temperature

As is the case for other impression materials, rubber base impression material is sensitive to the temperature at which it is mixed. The effect of temperature on rubber base material is as follows: The reaction rate will double with every 18°F increase in temperature between the temperatures of 68°F and 158°F; thus variations in environmental temperature markedly influence setting time. This factor should be remembered if the impressions are to be taken with rubber base material in the field during temperature extremes.

Control of the setting time of polysulfide rubber can be obtained by varying the temperature of the mixing pad or slab. This means of controlling the setting time can be best achieved if a glass slab is used because a glass slab can be heated or cooled much more easily than a pad of oiled paper. If retardation of the setting time is desired for one reason or another the temperature of the slab should be decreased but never to the dew point of the local environment for reasons described below. If an increase of the setting time is desired the temperature of the slab should be increased, but not to a point at which the material becomes set on the pad before it can be mixed properly and used.

Humidity

Unlike impression plaster and nonreversible alginate hydrocolloid, the setting reaction of rubber base impression material is accelerated by small amounts of water. Therefore, this impression material is not suitable for outdoor use when the humidity is extremely high or when it is raining. Although a high humidity will only cause a decrease in working time and the effect is not extreme, it can be enough to be annoying and result in a needless waste of material. If it is raining, even if the object of which the impression is taken is sheltered, the chance of contaminating the mix with water is great enough that the material should not be selected for a mix in that environment.

If, furthermore, in an attempt to increase the setting time the mixing slab is cooled to a point at or below the dew point, moisture will condense out of the air onto the slab, contaminating the mixture with moisture and resulting in a rapid acceleration of the setting time, and again possibly resulting in the needless waste of these relatively expensive materials.

Dimensional Stability

Polysulfide rubber base impression material has much greater dimensional stability than nonreversible alginate hydrocolloid material when rubber base material is confined in a tray; the percent of distortion after thirty minutes is .00 percent. The percent of distortion after three days when the material is confined to a tray is only .013 percent. Bear in mind, however, that all materials can and will change dimensionally with time, however slight the change.

Rubber base impression material has been shown to exhibit some thermal shrinkage with temperature change, although this factor limiting its dimensional stability has been shown to be prevented by the adhesion of the rubber material to the impression tray by the adhesive material (usually a liquid) which is included in the rubber base kit by the manufacturer. Rubber base impression material is among the most accurate of the impression materials we have at this time.

Availability and Storage

Polysulfide rubber base impression material is sold in kits containing one large tube of rubber base material, another tube of accelerator material, and a small jar of adhesive intended to coat the custom or stock tray so the material will adhere to the tray and not to the object of the impression.

Both the base material and accelerator material, provided they have been packaged properly, are not known to deteriorate in the tubes during storage and can be expected to have an indefinite shelf life.

Recently some rubber base impression materials have been introduced with chemicals other than lead peroxide as an accelerator. These materials are not recommended as they are more expensive, less accurate, more difficult to use, and deteriorate after a period of time on the shelf.

Techniques

To use polysulfide rubber base impression material, the following items of equipment are necessary:

1. Either a glass mixing slab with a thermometer imbedded in it or an oil paper mixing pad. An unoiled paper mixing pad should not be used as the rubber impression material will adhere to it and it will be impossible to obtain a proper mix of the material;

2. a flexible stainless steel spatula with rounded corners. The spatula should be at least three-fourths inch wide and six inches long and have a handle large enough to grasp comfortably with the entire hand;

3. either a custom impression tray or a stock plastic impression tray to carry the material to the object of which the impression is to be taken, as described in Chapter 8; and

4. appropriate polysulfide rubber ingredients.

Polysulfide rubber base impression material is prepared in the following manner:

1. If a glass slab is used, it should be cooled or warmed as neces-

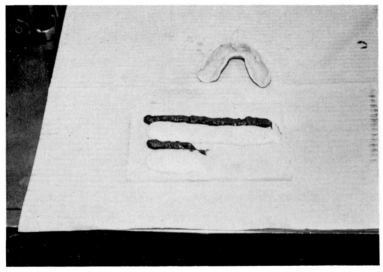

Figure 36. Polysulfide rubber base impression material on a waxed paper pad ready for mixing. The white material is the base paste; the dark material is the accelerator paste. An acrylic custom tray is shown at the top center of the illustration.

sary to compensate for environmental conditions.

2. Equal lengths of both accelerator paste and base paste should be squeezed onto the slab; the accelerator paste may be varied

as described in the section on base-accelerator ratio.

3. The blade of the flexible steel spatula should be coated completely on both sides with the accelerator material. Using the

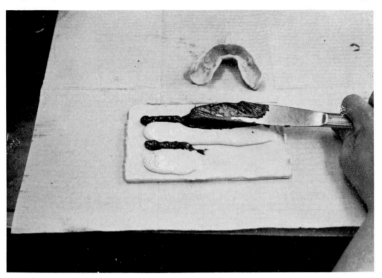

Figure 37. The spatula is coated with accelerator paste before mixing begins.

sharp edge of the blade of the spatula, the two ropes of the material should be combined with the first press of the spatula and the mixture should be mixed as directed by the manufacturer (about one minute), using a combined rotating and pressing motion.

4. When the material is completely mixed it should be of a uniform color; there should be no light streaks or dark areas. If light or dark streaks are present the materials have not been mixed adequately. A uniform texture is of utmost importance to an accurate impression, as the curing of a rubber base impression material will never be complete throughout the entire mass if the mixture is not completely homogeneous, and homogeneity is necessary to prevent distortions in the completed impression caused by collapsed air bubbles. Indentations may sometimes be found on the surfaces of impressions, appearing as nodules or round or half-round areas; this effect is due to the collapse of a void near the surface. If the material is mixed

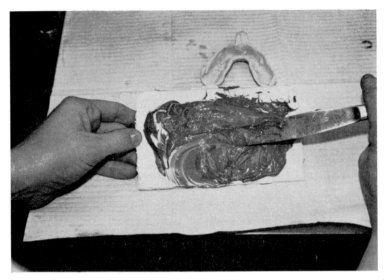

Figure 38. An incompletely mixed batch of polysulfide rubber base material. Note the light and dark streaks in the material.

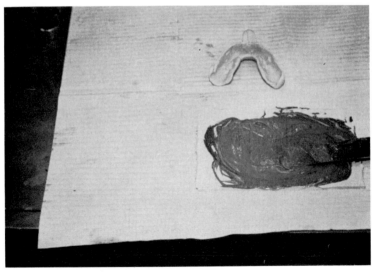

Figure 39. A completely mixed batch of polysulfide rubber base material. Note the even, uniform color.

    thoroughly and properly these bubbles will not be present.

5. Using the tip of the blade of the spatula, small amounts of the rubber base material should be placed quickly into whichever

type of tray is used. When the tray has been completely loaded the surface of the impression material should be gently

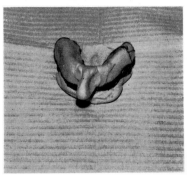

Figure 40. A custom tray filled with polysulfide rubber base material being used to duplicate a cast.

smoothed by the tip of the spatula and the tray should be carried smoothly against the object of which the impression is to be taken. The tray should be vibrated very gently as it is moved into place, then held firmly without motion until the material has set.

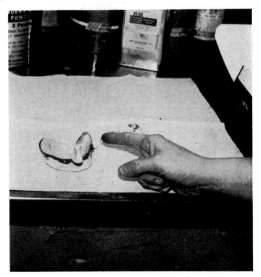

Figure 41. When the rubber base impression is stringy to the touch, the material has not set enough to allow removal of the impression.

6. The material should be checked by prodding it with a blunt instrument like a pencil tip. When the material is firm and returns to its original position quickly, leaving no depression, then the material has set enough to be removed. If the material is touched with a finger and it is no longer sticky this means that the vulcanization process is under way; it does not mean that the material is ready to be removed from the object. It is necessary to check it as described above.

7. The impression should be removed with a quick snap, as this

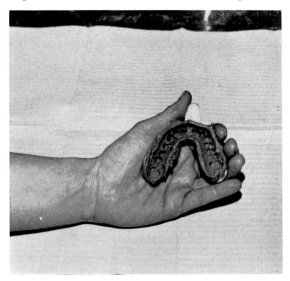

Figure 42. A completed polysulfide rubber base impression.

will cause the least distortion. If the type of plastic the custom tray is made from is a type of plastic which will soak up water from the environment with a resulting change in the dimensions of the tray itself, the impression should be stored in a dry place; otherwise a rubber base impression needs no special attention as an alginate impression does.

8. Upon written orders of a dentist, a cast should be made. Rubber base material has a much greater dimensional stability than alginate, but since it does continue to cure for as long as two days and may distort, as a general rule, impressions made from this material should be poured up within two or three hours of

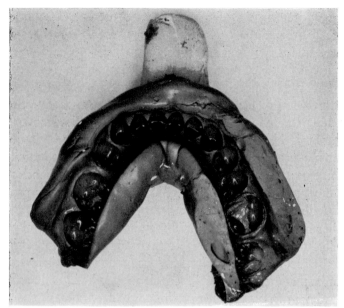

Figure 43. Closeup of a completed polysulfide rubber base impression. (Courtesy of E. H. Greener, et. al.: *Materials Science in Dentistry,* Baltimore, Wilkins, 1972, page 321.)

the time they are removed from the object.

9. Unlike plaster impression material and alginate hydrocolloid impression material, more than one cast may be poured from a rubber base impression material, providing the impression is cleaned adequately after being separated from the first cast. No more than three casts should be prepared from one impression. If more than these are prepared, the casts will be inaccurate because of the stresses and strains on the material by the repeated setting of a cast material and the repeated separation of the impression from the cast material. At least fifteen to thirty minutes should be allowed to lapse between the time of separation of the rubber base material from the object of the impression to allow for the phenomenon of a lasting return to compensate for minor areas of stretching in the impression as it is removed from the object and to allow for residual amounts of hydrogen gas produced by the curing reaction to dissipate.

Uses for Police

Polysulfide rubber base impression material is probably the most accurate impression material available for use in recording dental evidence. Its technique of preparation and use is relatively easy to learn; it is useful for the preparation of impressions capable of producing multiple casts; and it has an indefinite shelf life. Although rubber base impression material is more expensive than alginate impression material or impression plaster, it is less expensive than silicone rubber base impression material. Its primary disadvantage is the fact that it is highly sensitive to moisture contamination, which limits its use out of doors; and the setting reaction produces hydrogen sulfide gas, the odor of which resembles rotten eggs and is offensive to most people. The lead peroxide in the accelerator paste will cause indelible stains on clothing.

Rubber base impression material may be used as a general purpose impression material when extremely fine and accurate impressions are needed for record purposes. Impressions made with this material are so accurate that casts produced from them may be introduced as evidence and not merely used for preliminary analysis by the dentist. In cases where the dentist wishes for the purposes of analysis to have casts of extremely high quality, rubber base impression material is preferred. Rubber base impression material, as well as nonreversible alginate hydrocolloid, should be on hand in every criminology laboratory.

SILICONE RUBBER BASE IMPRESSION MATERIAL

Another type of synthetic rubber is one in which the polymer molecule is based on an organic silicone compound as opposed to the sulphur rubber compound of standard polysulfide rubber base material. Silicone base impression material, as it is commonly known, is similar to polysulfide rubber base impression material mainly in the fact that they are both rubber but in few other ways.

No specific analysis of silicone rubber impression material is available. However, most contain a base paste consisting of a silicone gum or proto form of rubber containing a-polydimethyl siloxane and a-polyethyl silicate. Both of these materials are in liquid form so a filler of silica is used to convert this material into a paste. Silicone base material vulcanizes in contact with a liquid accelerator compound containing an organic metal and some type of alkyl silicate.

The manufacture of the silicone rubber base impression material base paste is very difficult because the intermolecular attractions between the silicone polymers are much less than in other synthetic rubber compounds. So a filler must be selected which will not weaken the intermolecular attractions even further. The particle size of the individual pieces of the silica filler should be about the same as the size of the silicone polymer molecule; the average diameter of the particles may be as small as 10 to 20 μmm. The particle size also must not be too small or the filler may form into clumps or may separate. Because of these difficulties in manufacture, silicone impression material is more expensive than polysulfide rubber.

The accelerator liquid for silicone base impression material usually contains an organo-metal such as tin octoate or tin caprylate and a type of ethyl silicate. Because the setting reaction initiated by the tin octoate causes large amounts of hydrogen gas to be produced, the accelerator liquid also contains hydrogen acceptors such as analdehyde or chromium oxide or both. This material is not a catalyst and in no way enters into any of the chemical reactions resulting in the vulcanization of the silicone rubber material, but instead captures and binds the hydrogen molecules as the escaping gas is formed. The material, a compound of hydrogen and chromium oxide, becomes an integral part of the rubber material, not altering its physical properties significantly. The accelerator liquid is generally tinted a pastel color.

Variables

Silicone rubber base impression material is subject to variations of mixing time and setting time, and resulting changes in the accelerator-base ratio and temperature as follows:

Mixing Time

There is a considerable amount of variation in the time of mixing and setting of silicone rubber base impression material from manufacturer to manufacturer. The mixing time varies from approximately two minutes at 98.6°F to four minutes at 77°F and the setting time varies from three and one-half minutes at 98.6°F to over eight minutes at 77°F. The length of time the silicone impression material is mixed has little effect if any on the setting time.

Base-Accelerator Ratio

As is the case for polysulfide rubber base impression material, changes in the ratio of the accelerator liquid to the base paste will produce changes in the working and setting times of the silicone impression material. In fact, varying the ratio of accelerator liquid to base paste is about the only method available for controlling the mixing time and setting time of the silicone base material. It should be noted that it is easier to lengthen the mixing time and setting time by reducing the amount of accelerator used than it is to shorten the mixing and setting times by increasing the accelerator beyond a certain point. Attempts to control the setting time by diluting the accelerator with small amounts of commercially available liquid silicone chemicals prevents the silicone material from setting up at all, or at best leaves a sticky surface on the impression material.

Temperature

Unlike polysulfide rubber base material, temperature has apparently little effect on the setting time and mixing time and physical properties of silicone rubber base material. However, there is a sensitivity to temperature after the material has set up; the material has the property of thermal expansion as the temperature goes up or down.

Dimensional Stability

Although silicone rubber base impression material is far more stable dimensionally than nonreversible alginate hydrocolloid, it is less stable than polysulfide rubber base impression material for a number of reasons. Shrinkage over a period of time is more likely to occur because the process of curing takes longer in the case of silicone rubber than it does in the case of polysulfide rubber. Also the continued curing of the silicone base material after it has been removed from the mouth or other object results in the continued production of large amounts of hydrogen gas which produces a certain amount of shrinkage as a by-product of this chemical reaction. Additionally, silicone base impression material is subject to a condensation reaction which causes additional shrinkage. Finally, the dimensional stability of silicone base material is also sensitive to temperature, a disadvantage described above.

When confined to a tray, silicone rubber base impression material at the end of thirty minutes may show any kind of dimensional change from a shrinkage of 0.3 percent to an expansion of 0.5 percent. After three days, if confined to a tray, silicone rubber material may show anything from a shrinkage of .40 percent to an expansion of .13 percent. Therefore, the silicone is clearly not as stable as poly-sulfide rubber base impression material.

Availability and Storage

Silicone base impression material is supplied by the manufacturer in kits in one of two fashions: in the first instance the kit may include a tube containing the base paste and a small bottle containing the liquid accelerator and a third bottle containing the adhesive. Other manufacturers may supply the silicone base impression material in a kit containing a large metal drum of base paste, portions of which may be removed with a large spoon or a scoop, and containing a bottle of liquid accelerator compound and another bottle containing the tray adhesive.

Unlike rubber base impression material, silicone rubber base impression material does have a limited shelf life. The base material will stiffen with time, and the length of time the material can be stored and not lose its physical properties is no more than nine months. If the silicone paste is continually exposed to the air, the length of time it can be stored without permanent damage is shortened; so if the cap on the tube of the silicone base paste is not replaced or the lid of the base material drum is not quite closed, the material will stiffen and become useless in about three months.

The accelerator paste also deteriorates with age. Tin octoate is a very unstable material with a shelf life of only about five months. Under no circumstances should either the base paste or the accelerator compound ever be kept in a place where the temperature is higher than 80°F, and the longest shelf life will be obtained if they are kept in the refrigerator.

Because of this limited shelf life phenomenon, any time silicone base impression material is purchased it should be tested immediately to see whether the material is fresh or whether it has been on the shelf for a while. If the working time of the material is not in the range of three and one-half minutes and the setting time in the range of about seven minutes, if the paste is too stiff or sticky or if the accelerator liquid shows any signs of thickening or jelling the material should be returned for replacement.

Techniques

The materials needed to prepare silicone base impressions are the following:

1. an oil paper mixing pad. Standard unoiled paper should not be used as a mixing pad because the base material will adhere to it and be impossible to mix properly;
2. a flexible metal spatula with a flat end and rounded corners. The spatula should be at least three-fourths inch wide with a handle large enough to fit comfortably into the entire hand;
3. either a preformed stock or a custom impression tray to carry the material to the object of the impression, as described in Chapter 8; and
4. silicone impression material ingredients.

Mixing and utilization of silicone rubber base impression material should proceed as follows:

1. The desired amount of silicone base material should be placed on the mixing pad. If in a tube, the desired length of silicone base material should be squeezed from the tube onto the pad. If the silicone material is supplied in paste form in a drum, the desired number of scoops of base material should be carefully placed on the mixing pad.
2. The accelerator should be placed next. If the base material is supplied in a tube then one to two drops of accelerator liquid should be placed beside the rope of base material for each inch of base material. If the base material is supplied in a drum one to two drops of liquid accelerator are placed on each scoop of base.
3. The impression material should be stirred vigorously with rotating and pressing motions of the spatula until it is mixed, for a period of time not to exceed three and one-half minutes. When mixed the impression material should be of a uniform color with no streaking or changes and variations in color throughout the entire mass. The entire mass of material absolutely must be homogeneous. The result of a mixture that is not homogeneous will be the same as the result of this error with polysulfide rubber impression material, as described in Item 4 of techniques for handling polysulfide rubber impression material; namely, there will be distortions which could ruin the impression.
4. Using the edge of the spatula, small amounts of the impression material should be placed in the tray and the tray loaded in this

manner as quickly as possible. When the tray has been slightly overfilled it is ready to be placed into the mouth or against the object.

5. The tray of silicone impression material, if it is to be used inside the mouth, should be seated all the way using firm pressure and a gentle vibrating motion. If the object of the impression is outside the mouth the tray also should be seated against it firmly but gently with a slight vibrating motion. The tray should then be held motionless until the material sets.

6. The material should be checked periodically with a blunt instrument such as a pencil tip. When gentle pressure with a pencil tip no longer leaves an indentation in the impression material, the material is ready for removal. If the impression material is no longer sticky to the touch but light pressure still leaves an indentation, the material is curing but has not completely set. When the material no longer leaves an indentation when lightly touched with a pencil tip, the material should be removed quickly with a sharp, quick snap.

7. A cast should be made from the impression on orders of a dentist. Since large amounts of hydrogen gas are produced by the setting reaction of silicone impression material, thirty to forty-five minutes should be allowed to elapse before the impression is poured up with cast material in order to allow sufficient time for most of the hydrogen gas to be produced. However, no more than forty-five minutes should be allowed to pass before the silicone impression is poured up because of the relative lack of dimensional stability.

8. Like polysulfide rubber impression materials, more than one cast can be prepared from silicone base impression material impressions, assuming that the impression is properly cleaned after the impression is separated from the cast. However, no more than two casts should be prepared from a single impression.

Uses for Police

Silicone base impression material is another highly accurate impression material. Its accuracy is almost as great as polysulfide rubber base impression material, but it is much cleaner and more pleasant to use; it does not produce a disagreeable odor as it vulcanizes, and it does not stain clothing as does polysulfide rubber material. This impression material may be used as a general purpose impression material when extremely accurate models and casts are desired for analysis for the dentist or generally for making impressions of items of evidence.

Its disadvantages are its relatively high cost, the very short shelf life, and its relative dimensional instability in comparison with that of polysulfide rubber impression material. However, it is less affected by extremes of temperature and water contamination than polysulfide rubber impression material is.

On the balance, although both silicone rubber and polysulfide rubber base material are excellent for general use for taking impressions for legal purposes, the polysulfide rubber base impression material is the most useful. However, in cases when the disadvantages of silicone impression material can be overlooked, this accurate material is most serviceable and should be available for forensic purposes.

DENTAL WAX

Wax is used in the field of dental evidence for the purpose of ob-

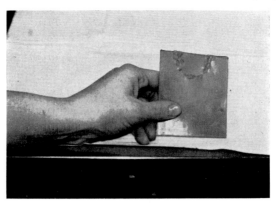

Figure 44. A wax bite registration showing the alignment of the subject's upper teeth.

taining what is called a bite registration. A bite registration is an impression of the biting surfaces of teeth in a piece of wax.

Wax

Wax is a polymer and occurs naturally in nature. Some types of wax, such as carnuba and cocoa butter, are made by plants; plant waxes generally are relatively solid and have a high melting point. Other waxes are made by insects, for example beeswax which is high in polyunsaturated carbons and hence has a low melting point. Still other waxes are mineral waxes, such as paraffin, which is derived from petroleum. And still other types of wax, such as castor wax, acrowax C and albacer, are man-made waxes; these waxes generally are derived from petroleum or petroleum products and are usually more flexible and more plastic-like than paraffin.

Most wax is chemically inert. Making a wax, whether artificially or in nature, involves a long, involved chain of chemical reactions, and by the time the final product is achieved, it is incapable of further chemical reactions.

The characteristics and physical properties of wax depends on the type of wax and upon the composition of the wax. The physical properties of wax depend on the strength of the chemical ties holding the molecules of the wax chain together, i.e. the stronger the chemical linkage, the more brittle the wax; the weaker the chemical linkage, the softer and more easily meltable is the wax. The presence of incidental impurities in wax also affects its physical properties. The more impurities in the wax, the less stable the wax is, and the softer and more plastic it is. Animal wax, such as beeswax, tends to have a relatively high percentage of impurities, hence tends to be softer.

Because natural waxes contain varying degrees of impurities, there is very little consistency in composition from one batch of wax to another; this can cause considerable problems in the working and manipulative properties of the wax. For this reason synthetic or artificial wax, where the composition is exact and controlled and hence more dependable, is being used more and more today in dentistry. Most wax used in industry is either synthetic wax or is wax made from two or more natural ingredients to which are added small amounts of materials such as synthetic waxes, oils and coloring agents.

Bite Registration Wax

The kind of wax used to take bite registrations is called bite registration wax. There are many different kinds of bite registration wax in use today, most of which contain beeswax along with a mineral wax such as paraffin and smaller amounts of coloring agents and stearic acid and resin. The combination of paraffin, beeswax, stearic acid and resin is intended to produce a wax which is relatively hard and firm at room temperature, but which is soft and pliable and capable of taking and holding an impression and exhibiting some properties of deformation and flow at mouth temperature (98.6°F). To this mixture are added large amounts of tiny filings of a metal, either silver or silver amalgam (a mixture of silver and mercury), or copper. One commonly used type of bite registration wax consists of two layers of a typical registration wax heavily impregnated with filings of copper, and sandwiching between them a sheet of copper foil or aluminum foil. To facilitate softening, the bite registration wax is occasionally heated gently before use, and the purpose of the metal filings is to distribute this heat evenly throughout the wax, to keep one portion of the wax from becoming hotter than another, resulting in a tendency to warp and flow out of proportion to itself.

Variables

All wax is greatly influenced by temperature. The other variables influencing impression materials do not apply here. At temperatures considerably below the point at which wax becomes a hard solid, it behaves as a very brittle material. However, the greater the temperature, the more elastic wax becomes, until it reaches a point at which it deforms readily. Any material, when it is deformed, has a tendency to return to its original condition. This tendency in wax depends on the internal molecular structure and some waxes deform more readily than others. However, all wax above a certain point tends to flow or melt and to reestablish itself in its new configuration upon cooling. Stresses created within the wax itself can be relieved. After the wax has been heated and the stresses relieved, the wax will tend to stay in its new position and will resist being moved away, and if moved away, will have a tendency to creep or flow back.

Most wax in general tends to expand upon heating by greater amounts than other materials. Because of the type of bonds which hold it together, synthetic waxes made from petroleum by-products tend to expand more per unit volume than plant or animal waxes do.

Dimensional Stability

Wax is not dimensionally stable. Temperature changes will cause wax to expand or to contract, to creep, flow or wilt. It is irrelevant to give specific figures as to degrees or percentages of expansion or contraction, flowing or wilting because this varies considerably with manufacturers, depending on the exact composition of the wax; what percentage is paraffin or beeswax, and what other components, such as particles of metal or other chemicals, may be present. The changes in the properties of the wax can even vary from one batch of wax to another when produced by the same manufacturer because of the variations in the composition. All that is important to know is that dental wax is not stable and should not be relied upon for any measurement of any importance without making other more accurate records.

Availability and Storage

Bite registration wax is available at all dental supply houses, and is sold in boxes generally of ten to fifty sheets or wafers. Care should be taken to obtain a type of wax impregnated with metal chips rather than simply beeswax or beeswax and paraffin mixtures.

Storage of wax is no particular problem, and it may be stored at room temperature.

Techniques

Using bite registration wax, the technique of taking a bite registration is as follows:

1. A wax wafer approximately the size of the dental arch covering a line from the farthest back tooth on one side to the farthest back tooth on the other, or the position that would normally be occupied by the farthest back tooth on the other, should be selected.
2. The wax wafer should be trimmed with a pair of scissors so that it does not extend beyond the position of the farthest back tooth on either side.
3. Using either an open flame from an alcohol torch or hot water, the wax should be heated until it becomes soft.
4. The softened wax-metal sandwich should then be placed gently on the lower teeth in contact with all the lower teeth.
5. The subject should be asked to run the tip of his tongue around all of the surfaces of the upper teeth to moisten them gently. He should then bite down and try to bite all of the way through the wax sandwich on both sides while his tongue is

placed as far back as possible on the roof of his mouth. The subject should maintain a hard, firm biting pressure for a period of three minutes.

6. After three minutes have elapsed, the subject should be told to open his mouth very quickly. This will separate one-half of the teeth, usually the upper, from the wax bite registration.

7. Using a sharp pointed tip such as a dental explorer or a probe, the operator should gently tease the wax bite registration off the lower teeth, beginning with the back teeth on one side and then on the other. When the wax bite registration has been loosened from all sections of the mouth, it should be carefully and gingerly removed from the teeth and immediately placed in a bowl of cold water.

8. This procedure should be repeated at least twice, producing a total of three bite registrations.

9. After the three bite registrations have been taken, one should be kept on file as a negative record of the imprint left of the individual's bite; the second registration should be used as an aid in positioning the upper and lower casts of the subject in

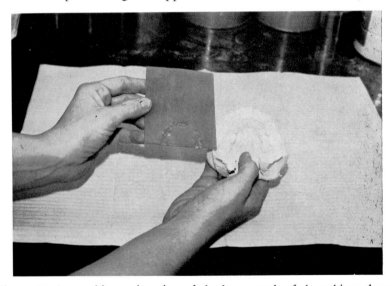

Figure 45. A wax bite registration of the lower arch of the subject shown beside an accurate cast of the subject's lower teeth. In this picture the right side of the wax bite corresponds to the left side of the dental cast.

their proper relation to each other; and the third bite registration should have casts prepared of the imprints on both sides using techniques to be described in Chapter 7 on the orders of a dentist.

Uses for Police

Dental bite registration wax is used in dental evidence work for the purpose of obtaining a record of the types of marks or imprints left by the subject as he bites into an object. This is necessary supportive evidence and is intended for comparison with the photographs and casts of impressions of the original bite marks, or occasionally for experimental duplication of the bite mark or pattern on an instrument called an articulator. This is valuable supportive evidence, but should never be relied upon as a sole record of the bite mark.

Chapter 7 __ __ __ __ __ __ __ __ __

CAST MATERIALS AND TECHNIQUES

__ __ __ __ __ __ __ __ __ __ __ __

CASTS ARE CONSTRUCTED from impressions and are the purpose for which impressions are made. Accurate casts are records of the mouth used by the dentist in making comparisons and judgments about the dental evidence at hand.

There are two ways the police may obtain casts. One way is to send the impressions to a dental laboratory where they will be poured up into casts. This may be cheaper in the short run or instances where the department has only a very few cases, and even then it is only possible if impression materials are used which can last until they arrive at the laboratory and are poured up. In cases when it is essential to prepare the cast within only a few minutes, the police department should have available the materials and the trained person who can make the cast. Reference should be made to Chapter 6 for specific amounts of time available between removing the impression and the necessary time to make the cast and fit this information to individual circumstances.

The second way for police to obtain casts is to make them all themselves. The initial cost of the materials and equipment is higher than sending them out, but will result in eventual savings for the department, particularly the large department. Needless to say, this is also the most convenient way, and some large metropolitan areas or states may wish to set up one laboratory for many jurisdictions. In any case, it is necessary to have at least enough equipment and materials for some cases, and the department should develop a working relationship with a dental laboratory, with the assistance of the department's dentist, for those it chooses not to do itself.

According to the Dental Practice Act, it is absolutely necessary to submit impressions for cast construction along with a *written* work order signed by a licensed dentist. This is true if the cast is made in the police department laboratory as well as if it is sent to an outside laboratory. Therefore, the police should make sure they have the written work order signed by the dentist before proceeding. In all states, persons designated as technicians or assistants working under the direct guidance and supervision of a licensed dentist may construct casts from impressions, although in these cases a *pro forma* work authorization is necessary.

Regardless of the department's choice whether or not to do all the casts themselves, it is necessary for the police to know the scientific information about the materials discussed in this chapter, particularly acrylic because acrylic is necessary for the construction of custom trays for taking certain types of impressions.

PLASTERS FOR CASTS
DENTAL STONE

The physical and chemical aspects of dental plaster have already been discussed in Chapter 6 in the portion of the impression plaster section dealing with plaster in general. Dental stone sets by the same mechanisms as other plaster, including dental impression plaster. The ingredients which go into making dental stone commercially are basically the same ingredients which go into making an impression plaster, with the notable exception that dental stone does not contain a material such as cornstarch or potato starch to weaken it. The characteristics of dental stone are affected by the same factors which affect the physical properties of impression plaster.

Dental stone differs from the dental impression plaster only in the way in which it is manufactured and in the strength of the set product. Dental stones are made by heating the refined gypsum to temperatures of 253.4°F in a piece of equipment called an autoclave under steam pressure equaling seventeen pounds per square inch for a period of four to five hours. This produces a type of plaster where the particles consist of very thin, needle-like crystals which are smaller than the larger, irregularly shaped crystals found in plaster of paris. These thin, needle-like crystals also contain much less water in the crystal structure than the larger crystals found in plaster of paris. When mixed with water and the mixture is allowed to set the thin, needle-like crystals produce a set product which is much more dense and much less porous than plaster of paris.

Variables

Dental stone is affected by variations in mixing time, water-powder ratio, temperature, and added accelerators and retarders, as described below. Since this material is a plaster, information included in the section dealing with plaster in general in Chapter 6 is not duplicated, only amended as necessary to this particular variation of the material, and reference should be made to that section for complete information.

Mixing Time

The effects of variations in mixing time on dental stone are the same as the effects of variations in mixing time on the properties of impression plaster.

Water-Powder Ratio

The effects of variations of the water-powder ratio on the setting reaction and physical properties of dental stone are basically the same as the effects of the variations of the water-powder ratio on the physical properties and setting reaction of dental impression plaster. However, dental stone requires much less water to make a workable mixture than dental impression plaster or plaster of paris does. While most plasters require a W/P ratio of 0.3 to 0.5, most dental stones have a W/P ratio in the range of 0.2 to 0.25.

Temperature

The effects of variations in temperature in the water used for mixing plaster and in the environmental temperature produce the same changes and effects in the setting reactions and physical properties of dental stone as they do in the case of dental impression plaster.

Accelerators

As mentioned in the previous chapter, accelerator chemicals are the most reliable way to control the setting time of plaster. As with dental impression plaster, potassium sulfate is most often used, but table salt in the concentration of one tablespoon per one pint of water used to mix plaster will also produce an acceleration of the setting time.

As is the case with impression plaster, accelerators have an effect on setting and expansion. The worst offender in this respect is terra alba; plasters with this as an accelerator compound should be avoided as a material to record evidence.

Retarders

As described in Chapter 6, a retarder is a chemical added to plaster powder with the purpose of slowing the setting time. As is the case with dental impression plaster, the most commonly used retarders are borax and sodium citrate. Some dental stones do contain small amounts of retarders to act along with the accelerator to produce a finer control over the setting time, although the amount of the retarders used and their effect on the setting reaction and setting time and expansion of dental stone used in the preparation of dental casts is negligible. The concern here is primarily not with lengthening the setting time but with shortening it.

Dimensional Stability

All plasters do expand somewhat on setting. However, the expansion of dental stone is in the range of from 0.05 percent to 0.10 percent, an amount of expansion which is negligible for purposes in this field.

Availability and Storage

Dental stone is sold in containers of from one to fifty pounds, available at a dental supply house. Since it is used in fairly large quantities, it is most economical to purchase the larger containers of this material.

The dental stone container should be kept tightly sealed so that moisture in the air will not cause it to start to set. The temperature at which it is stored is not important, and it may be stored at room temperature.

Techniques

The following items of equipment and materials are needed to prepare and use dental stone:

1. a round, flexible rubber bowl of a size that will fit comfortably in the hand;
2. a stiff-bladed metal spatula. The blade of the spatula should be three-fourths inch to one inch wide and stiff, because a flexible blade will drag as it moves through a thick mixture of dental stone resulting in a mixture which is not thorough. The

end of the spatula should be rounded at the corners so that it will conform to the shape of the inside of the bowl. If a square-bladed spatula is used, areas along the surface of the bowl will not be touched with the spatula and the mixing will not be complete;

3. a scale for measuring powder and a measuring device for water;

4. a glass slab or linoleum pad;

5. dental stone plaster material;

6. an automatic vibrator, which is basically a small electrical engine with an eccentric wheel attached to a platform. As the motor runs, the eccentric wheel turns causing the platform to vibrate; this aids in the expulsion of air bubbles from a mixture of plaster which is placed upon it;

7. a mechanical spatulator (optional) consisting of a flexible rubber bowl, a metal cover to the center of which metal cover is attached a two to three-blade rotor with a handle. This machine is intended to produce a smoother and better mix of plaster with fewer bubbles;

8. a vacuum spatulator (optional) consisting of a plastic container with a rotor in the center of a plastic cap to which are attached metal blades. An attachment coming out of the plastic cap allows a hose to be affixed, the other end of which is joined to a small motor producing a vacuum. The motor which produces the vacuum also has an attachment connected to the same shaft as the blades, causing them to rotate very rapidly. As the blades are rotating and the stone is mixed, the vacuum engine is removing the air from the plaster bowl to prevent the formation of bubbles. An airtight rubber seal around the edge of the lid insures that no additional air enters to replace the air being removed;

9. a model trimmer (optional). This is basically an electric engine attached to a large rotary wheel embedded with industrial-grade garnets or powdered carborundum, which is used to trim the bases or edges of a cast so they present a uniform and pleasing appearance.

The following procedures should be performed to result in properly mixed and used dental stone:

1. The proper amount of water should be measured and poured either into the mixing bowl, the mechanical spatulator, or the bowl of the vacuum spatulator.
2. To this water the proper amount of plaster for the desired water-powder ratio should be added slowly.
3. The mixture of plaster should be stirred vigorously until the mixture is smooth and homogeneous. If a mechanical spatulator is used it should preferably be placed on a vibrator and the lid should be held down tightly while the crank handle is turned as rapidly as possible for at least one minute and preferably two to three minutes. If a vacuum spatulator is used the lid should be sealed in place, the vacuum hose hooked up, the electric motor turned on and the shaft the blades are attached to joined to the fitting on the outside of the electric engine causing it to rotate very rapidly. This should be done for between one and two minutes.
4. The impression to be filled with dental stone is placed on the edge of the mechanical vibrator, and the mechanical vibrator is turned on. Using the end of the spatula, very small amounts of plaster are lifted from the bowl (or the mechanical spatu-

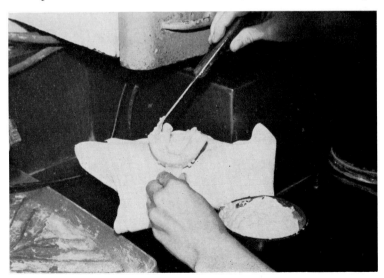

Figure 46. Pouring dental stone into an impression, the first step in constructing a cast.

lator or the vacuum spatulator) and placed at the back of the impression and the impression held so that the mix of stone will slowly be vibrated down into the farthest recesses of the impression. This action is repeated again and again until the entire impression is filled with dental stone to overflowing.

5. The excess stone is placed either on the linoleum pad or glass

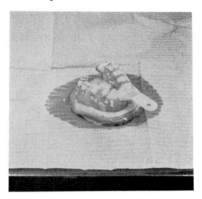

Figure 47. A common mistake: the paper this newly poured stone cast has been placed on to set up is leaching water from the mix of stone. This will affect the properties of the stone in a negative way.

slab and a small mound is formed. On the top of this mound the filled impression should be inverted so that the plaster filling the impression contacts the plaster mound.

6. Using the edge of the spatula, the plaster of the mound on the glass slab should be blended with the plaster in the impression.

7. The plaster should be allowed to sit undisturbed until its setting reaction has been completed, a process which normally occurs in thirty to forty-five minutes; when set, the plaster no longer feels warm to the touch.

8. When the plaster has completely set, the impression may be separated from the set mix of stone. First a pocket knife should be used to carefully remove what small chips of stone may overlap onto the tray preventing its easy separation. Then carefully, the tray with the impression material should be re-

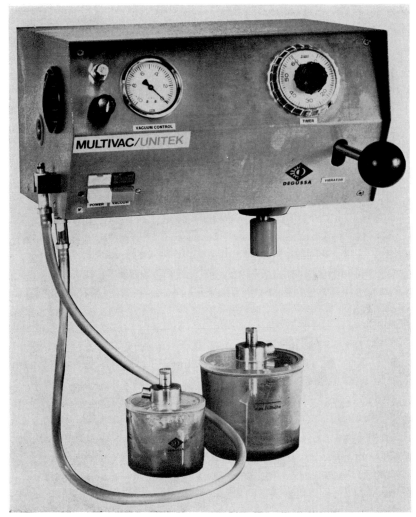

Figure 48. A vacuum spatulator used to mix dental stone without incorporating bubbles in it. (Courtesy of Unitek Corporation, Monrovia, California.)

moved upwards, away from the cast material with as quick but smooth a motion as possible, and with support of the base of the cast as it is done.

9. The finished set stone cast should be taken to the model trimmer, and there, with care so none of the important areas of the cast are touched, the edges of the cast should be trimmed to present a smooth and uniform appearance.

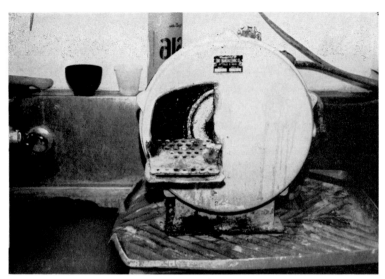

Figure 49. A model trimmer, used to trim the bases of stone casts.

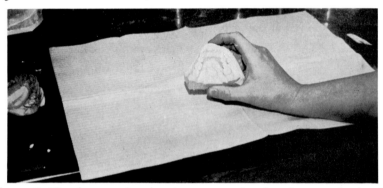

Figure 50. The first step in trimming a cast, trimming the posterior border of the cast.

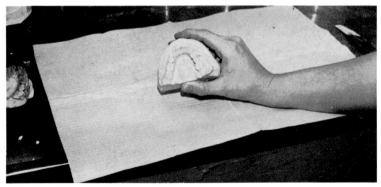

Figure 51. The second step in trimming a cast, trimming the sides of the cast. The front edge will be trimmed next.

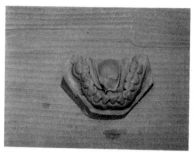

Figure 52. A freshly trimmed cast. Note the unusual alignment of the front teeth; these teeth would leave a very distinctive bite mark.

Uses for Police

Dental stone is a good all around material for the construction of casts of both the teeth and other parts of the body and items of physical evidence for both analysis and for record purposes. It is reasonably accurate, dimensionally stable, durable, and the techniques of manipulation are relatively easy to learn. There are very few instances when this material will not be satisfactory, both for purposes of analysis and for purposes of records.

DIE STONE CAST MATERIAL

Die stone is basically a very strong dental stone. Whereas most dental stone withstands pressures of 5,000 to 6,000 pounds per square inch, die stone will withstand pressures in the range of 8,000 to 9,000 pounds per square inch. Since die stone is essentially a very strong dental stone and shares in minute detail most of the physical properties and setting reactions of dental stone and is manufactured in the same way, this material will not be described in much detail.

Variables

Die stone is affected by the same variables in the same manner as is dental stone, with the only significant difference being in the water-powder ratio. The variables applicable to both dental stone and die stone of mixing time, water-powder ratio, temperature and retarders and accelerators are compared below.

Mixing Time

The variations in mixing time affect the mix and the setting of die stone in exactly the same way that variations of mixing time affect dental stone.

Water-Powder (W/P) Ratio

Die stone requires a much lower water-powder ratio than is used with dental stone to produce a workable mix. Die stone should be mixed with a W/P ratio of 0.15 to 0.20.

Temperature

Changes in temperature in both the water and the environment affect the setting and the physical properties of die stone in the same manner as they affect the properties of dental stone.

Retarders and Accelerators

The same retarders and accelerators are used in die stone as are used in dental stone and impression plaster, as described earlier in this chapter and in the beginning of Chapter 6.

Dimensional Stability

The dimensional stability of die stone is much greater than that of dental stone. The linear expansion of die stone is in the range of 0.07 percent to 0.10 percent and it has a volumetric contraction of approximately 4 percent.

Availability and Storage

Die stone may be purchased from any dental supply house, and is generally sold in containers containing from one-half pound to five pounds, smaller amounts than in many other bulk containers of dental materials. Because of the very low water-powder ratio needed to mix this material, a little bit goes a long way, and it is not necessary to buy very large quantities of this material at a given time.

As is the case for all plaster products, die stone should be stored in a container that is very tightly closed to prevent the die stone from absorbing moisture from the air, thus initiating a setting reaction which could destroy the working properties of the material.

Techniques

All of the techniques of preparation and mixing and all of the materials needed for preparation and mixing of die stone are the same as those needed for dental stone, with two exceptions:

1. Die stone must be mixed with extra care because it is a much thicker material, and thus there is a greater likelihood of inadvertently stirring air bubbles into the mixture, and
2. die stone must be vibrated much more than dental stone must be when pouring it into an impression because of its thickness and the likelihood of inadvertently incorporating air bubbles into the mix.

Uses for Police

Die stone is the preferred material when an extremely accurate cast is required for analysis and presentation of evidence.

ACRYLIC CAST MATERIAL

Acrylic is the name given to a type of plastic. The general term *plastic* encompasses a vast spectrum of materials, some of which resemble rubber, others are hard and firm, still others appear to be made of fibers, and some can actually be woven as cloth. All plastics are alike in that they are made up of giant molecules containing long and complex chains of smaller molecules. The properties and characteristics of each type of plastic is determined by the type and form of each individual type of plastic molecule.

Plastic is a nonmetal synthetic material, artificially formed from other materials which contain large amounts of carbon. Molecules of these other substances containing carbon are formed into long chains of giant molecules which determine the properties of the synthetic plastic. The plastic can generally be molded or poured into any form or shape desired.

Acrylic plastic material is one type of large synthetic plastic molecules. Acrylic is in the ethyline family of organic chemicals and is immediately derived from methacrylic acid, which is an organic compound that forms long chains through complicated chemical reactions which are beyond the scope of this book. There are two types of methacrylate (a synonym of acrylic): one is methyl-methacrylate and the other is ethyl-methacrylate, which differ in the number of carbons and some other atoms in the chain.

When acrylic plastics were first introduced, methyl-methacrylate was difficult and impractical to use. Elaborate and expensive equipment was needed to heat the plastic until it was softened. Then the material had to be injected into a mold contained in heated flasks under hydraulic pressure. During the 1930's it was discovered that it is possible to mix a powdered form of methyl-methacrylate with a liquid which simply contains a solution of the basic molecule of acrylic acid from which the acrylic polymer chain molecule is made, resulting in a dough which can then be packed into a mold and changed into the solid plastic by placing the mold under pressure and carefully heating it. This type of powder-liquid system is the same one we use today, with variations in the solidifying process. The ethyl-methacrylates were developed later and have been on the market only in recent years.

The plastic powder component is called the polymer, and the liquid component which contains simple acrylic acid is called the monomer. The polymer phase powder is composed of tiny, round plastic beads, the color of which is determined by the color of the inert and nonreactive pigment added to the plastic beads. It is possible to obtain commercial acrylics in just about any color imaginable; generally no other ingredients are added to the polymer phase besides coloring pigments.

The monomer liquid consists of a solution of alginic acid, to which is usually added a tiny amount (0.006% or less) of hydroquinone to prevent the monomer from curing and becoming solid when stored over a long period of time.

Today acrylics are categorized into two general types according to their setting reaction. These two types are the heat-cure acrylics and the self-cure (or cold cure) acrylics. The only difference between these acrylics is that the monomer phase of the self-cure acrylics contains a chemical which starts a chain of chemical reactions which results in the entire mixture turning into a solid mass of set methyl-methacrylate plastic. The heat-cure acrylics do not contain this accelerator and will not cure, for all practical purposes, unless they are heated to temperatures around 212°F for several hours.

Another type of acrylic, which has some uses in dental evidence, is the so-called soft acrylic. Soft acrylic is ordinary methyl-methacrylate which has had additional chemicals added to the monomer liquid which keeps the setting reaction from going all of the way to its completion, so that the final mass of plastic when it is set is soft and rubber-like, instead of firm and hard. Soft acrylics may be either heat-cure or cold-cure.

All acrylics set by an interesting process. Whether the acrylic used is a heat-cure acrylic or a self-cure acrylic, the basic process is the same and occurs in three stages. In the first stage, when the polymer is mixed with the monomer and a fluid mixture is formed, the monomer attacks the surface of the tiny beads of plastic polymer and penetrates these beads. The layer of polymer which has been attacked dissolves into the plastic solution and is dispersed throughout. The plastic becomes tacky and stringy to the touch. In the second stage, when the monomer has diffused into the polymer particles and as the mass of plastic becomes more saturated with polymer in solution and more layers of polymer are dissolved from the surface of these beads, the mixture becomes smooth and dough-like and is no longer sticky. This is called the dough or jell stage. When the material is in this stage, it may be packed, molded or flowed into any shape desired. In the third stage, the material sets and becomes very hard, giving off a considerable amount of heat in the process. This is one reason why the material is *never* used for impressions. The heat used by the setting reaction is great enough to literally cook human tissue and cause it to slough.

Variables

Acrylics are subject to variations in powder-liquid ratio and temperature as described below:

Mixing Time

The properties of methyl-methacrylate and ethyl-methacrylate acrylics are not appreciably affected by variations in mixing time.

Powder-Liquid Ratio

All acrylics have a definite powder-liquid ratio which should never be varied. If the amount of liquid monomer in proportion to the amount of solid powder polymer is varied so that too much liquid is used, the material will set only very slowly and over a long period of time, and the material will be very weak and dimensionally unstable. If too much powder polymer is used in proportion to the amount of liquid monomer present, parts of the material will set up rapidly and other parts will not set up at all, and the mixture will be shot through with porosities.

Temperature

Changes in temperature affect all acrylics in the following manner: The higher the environmental temperature in which a cold-cure acrylic is mixed, the faster the acrylic will set up. The environmental temperature during setting is obviously crucial for heat-cure acrylic; the higher the temperature the faster it will set, up to the point where the monomer starts to boil. This causes porosities and should be prevented.

Dimensional Stability

All types of acrylic are dimensionally unstable. All acrylics, whether self-cure or heat-cure, expand and distort by soaking up water from the air during high humidity. In the opposite manner, when acrylics are dried out or exposed to dry atmospheres for long periods of time they shrink. Both expansion and shrinkage produce warpage in the material. The setting reaction itself produces a large amount of heat and the material also warps from this cause as the material sets.

Availability and Storage

Acrylic is sold in kits containing a large bottle of tiny polymer beads (appearing as powder) and another bottle of monomer liquid. Some kits also contain mixing spatulas and mixing cups coated with an inert material, usually wax. Some kits contain covered glass jars in which the acrylic is to be mixed. All acrylic kits contain measures to assist in obtaining the proper ratio between liquid and powder phases.

Acrylic liquid should always be stored in a cool place. If the monomer is stored in a place where the temperature is more than 80°F, it will begin to thicken and gel in a period of time ranging from six months to two years. If stored in a cool place (70°F or less), or for best results in a refrigerator, the monomer will have an indefinite shelf life. The polymer or bead phase has an indefinite shelf life, will not set, and may be stored under any temperature conditions within reason.

Techniques

Both cold-cure or self-cure acrylic and heat-cure acrylic in both the regular hard and in the soft-cure forms have a use in dental evidence work, as will be shown later. The techniques for making casts of any acrylic are too complicated and the equipment in the case of heat-cure acrylic is too expensive to reasonably be performed and used in any police department, although this is definitely a cast material. All casts should be made at a dental laboratory equipped to construct these types of casts upon written orders of a licensed dentist. The police will have a definite and important use for cold-cure acrylic cast material in the construction of custom trays.

Prior to use, it is important to note the following precautions:

1. Acrylics should *never* be allowed to set up in contact with human tissue. All self-cure acrylics, with the exception of one type, called reline acrylic which has no use in dental evidence, are capable of setting up when in contact with human tissue, and give off a great amount of heat as the setting reaction progresses. The amount of heat given off is enough to cause blistering and serious burning if used on the skin, and blistering and serious burning and the resulting slough of all tissues with which the material is in contact down to the bone if the material is allowed to set to completion in the mouth.

2. Care should be taken that no one breathes the acrylic monomer fumes. The fumes of acrylic acid of the monomer liquid have been demonstrated to be fatal under certain conditions if breathed directly for any period of time. Therefore, the material should be used in a well-ventilated place, and the officer should be careful that he or anyone else in the vicinity where the acrylic is being used does not inhale the fumes of the monomer liquid. In some cases where this precaution has not been followed, fatalities have resulted.

Following is a description of the materials needed for mixing and using cold-cure acrylic:

1. a small porcelain or glass container with a lid in which to mix the material;

2. a small mixing spatula with rounded ends and a flat blade; the blade may or may not be flexible and should be no more than one-fourth inch wide at its widest point;

3. an eyedropper;

4. a measuring device to measure the proper amount of polymer

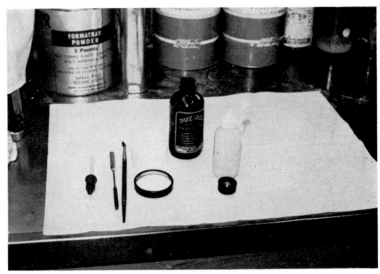

Figure 53. The setup of equipment needed to mix cold-cure acrylic.

and another to measure the proper amount of monomer; and
5. bottles of acrylic monomer and polymer ingredients.

The cold-cure acrylic should be prepared for use in a custom tray in the following manner:

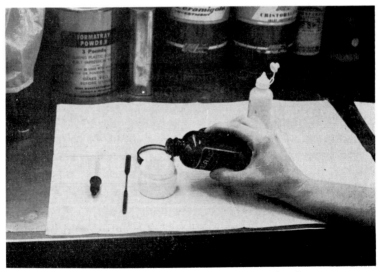

Figure 54. Cold cure monomer is poured into the mixing jar.

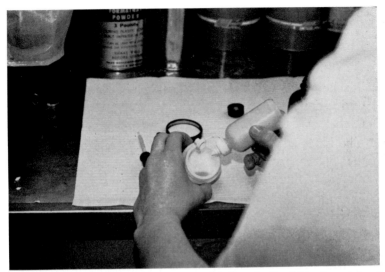

Figure 55. Cold cure polymer beads are added to the liquid in the mixing jar.

1. The desired amount of monomer liquid should be measured with the liquid measure and poured into the glass or ceramic or porcelain container.

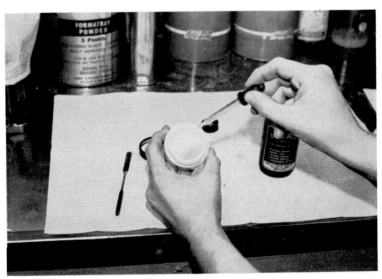

Figure 56. An extra drop of cold cure monomer is added just prior to mixing the cold cure acrylic.

2. To this liquid, the premeasured plastic polymer beads (or powder) should be slowly added until all of the liquid is absorbed and there is a fine layer of dry powder on top of the entire mass.

3. The container with the mass of acrylic inside should be turned upside down and tapped two or three times on a firm object to shake off the excess powder.

4. The batch of plastic is still too dry to use, so to this with the eyedropper should be added one or two drops of the monomer liquid.

5. The mixture should be vigorously stirred with the spatula until it reaches a smooth, homogeneous consistency, and with care not to include air bubbles in the mixture. If the mixture is stirred until it begins to become stringy, it should be thrown away since it has been mixed too long and the setting reaction has begun, which will be carried rapidly to completion.

6. Once the plastic mass has reached a smooth consistency and is not yet stringy, a tight cover should be placed over the glass or porcelain mixing jar and at one-minute intervals the jar should be opened and the surface should be touched with fingers. When the fingers are pulled away, if tiny amounts of the plastic stick to the fingers and form little strings as the

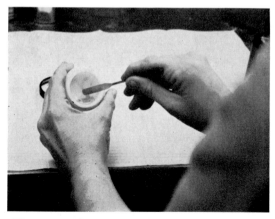

Figure 57. The acrylic is stirred with a small spatula.

fingers are pulled from the plastic mass, the plastic is not yet ready to use. When the plastic can be touched with the finger without removing bits of the plastic as the finger is pulled away, and when the plastic feels putty-like, it is ready to use.

7. Using the end of the spatula, the entire mass of plastic may be removed from the container. There is now approximately two minutes during which the plastic can be molded and formed into almost any shape desired before the setting re-

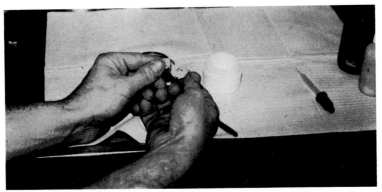

Figure 58. The acrylic is not ready to use when it is soft and crumbly.

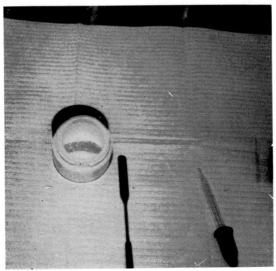

Figure 59. A small rope of doughlike acrylic ready to use.

action begins and the material can no longer be manipulated. It may now be used by police in making custom trays.

Uses for Police

Acrylic casts are only occasionally used in the field of dental evidence. Heat-cure acrylics are used in dental evidence in the construction of demonstration models and are especially good for this because their color is generally more life-like than the color which can be obtained with the cold-cure materials. There is also a type of soft heat-cure acrylic polymer, which, when processed, will have a soft and rubbery feel resembling soft rubber or with a little bit of imagination, human tissue, and is especially good for showing in public relations displays and table clinics (professional demonstrations), especially when the model depicts something with tissue laceration. There are also some models for this purpose constructed from cold-cure acrylic. Models are used where a high degree of realism is desired, and primarily in the following three instances:

1. for display purposes;
2. as models to be used for educational purposes in seminars or training sessions, and
3. for models to show to a jury when these realistic although dimensionally inaccurate models are requested by the attorney along with the primary impressions in a more standard material upon which the actual measurements were made.

Because of its extreme dimensional instability, acrylic should never be used as a cast material except for these purposes, and then only after primary accurate models have been obtained in other, more accurate, material. In any case, although they may be desirable to obtain, the police need not and should not attempt to make acrylic casts themselves, but should have them made when necessary at a properly equipped dental laboratory, accompanied by a written work order from a licensed dentist.

The biggest single use of acrylics in dental evidence work is for the construction and reinforcement of custom trays for use in taking some types of impressions, whether the impression is to be of an object, a part of the body or of the mouth. For this they are indispensable. Acrylics are used to construct custom trays in which highly accurate polysulfide or silicone impressions are taken, and their strength is crucial to a good impression. The techniques of preparation of a custom tray with this material are simple and are described in Chapter 8. Acrylics are also used to reinforce the edges of wire or perforated metal custom trays intended for taking impressions of parts of the body or of items of physical evidence with alginate impression material. The acrylic is placed around the edge of the tray to reinforce the tray and prevent the tray from warping and is used to construct a handle for the custom tray, all of which is described in detail in Chapter 8. The acrylic used for custom trays or for the reinforcement of metal custom trays is of the cold-cure variety.

ELECTROPLATING

Electroplating is a technique used to produce metal-covered casts. A polysulfide rubber impression is coated with either silver or copper powder, known as metalizer, and is placed into an electroplating solution containing a high concentration of either silver or copper molecules. Through this an electric current is run by positive and negative wires attached to an electrical unit. After a time, the metal becomes coated onto the impression. Cast material may be poured into this impression, and when the impression is removed, the metal will be attached to the cast, resulting in a very exact record of the object of the impression.

Variables

Electroplating is generally not subject to the same variables other cast materials are subject to and have only a few variables affecting the procedure and materials as follows:

Powder Coating

Only a uniform and light amount of metal powder should be placed upon the impression. A heavy coating will cause the material to crumble off.

Temperature and Light

The copper and silver metalized powder break down slowly during storage in all cases, but exposure to heat and light accelerate the process.

Dimensional Stability

Electroplate is extremely dimensionally stable, so no consideration of this is necessary in storage of the cast.

Availability and Storage

Electroplating units and the electroplating baths consisting of the metalizer and solution may be purchased from any dental supply house. However, anyone with a little electrical aptitude, such as the department's electrician, can manufacture a workable electroplating unit easily and much more inexpensively than one can be obtained from a supply house. The unit will be described in more detail under techniques.

The only two precautions which need to be taken with regard to the storage of materials used in the electroplating is to keep the bottles containing the silver or copper metalizer tightly closed to prevent tarnishing, although some of this will occur unavoidably, and the bottles containing the electroplating solution should be stored in a cool, dark place. Due to the inherent stability of these materials, no other precautions generally need be taken.

Techniques

To produce a metal-plated cast, the following materials are needed:

1. a polysulfide rubber base impression;
2. a large plastic container;
3. a jar of fine powdered silver or copper, called the metalizer;
4. a solution containing a high concentration of either silver or copper molecules, depending on whether the choice is silver plating or copper plating;
5. an electrical unit to which wires can be attached which in turn can be attached to the metalized portion of the impression. There are a number of different types of electroplating units designed for dental use which may be purchased from dental supply houses, each varying slightly according to the manufacturer; but all electroplating units contain the following elements: they all have a transformer (a device to reduce the line voltage); and a rectifier (a device to convert alternating current to direct current, necessary for electroplating); attachments which make it possible to adjust the amount of current; usually a meter to register the current reading of each setting; an on-off switch, a fuse, and the necessary dials;
6. two wires, at least one foot long, or long enough to reach

from the unit into the impression immersed in the bottom of the solution containing the metal molecules in the large plastic container;

7. A fine camelhair brush.

The following steps must be followed to produce an electroplated cast:

1. The polysulfide rubber impression should be dried carefully by blowing on it or patting it lightly with a soft paper towel. (A silicone impression may be used, but the results are not as good.)

2. With the fine camelhair brush, small amounts of the fine powdered silver or copper should be painted over all the surfaces of the impression to be electroplated. This is called *metalizing*.

3. The large plastic container should be filled to within an inch of the top with the solution of chemicals containing the high concentration of either silver or copper.

4. The wires should be attached to the positive and negative electrodes on the electroplating unit.

5. The terminal one-fourth inch of both the positive and negative wire leads should have the insulation scraped off. The ends of the wire which have the insulation scraped off should be inserted directly into the rubber impression material in noncritical areas. The wire should be inserted into the impression to the point where the impression and the insulation are actually in contact and into the metalized area.

6. The metalized impression with the wires attached should be placed into the plastic container with the plating solution in a position assuring that the entire impression is covered with the plating solution.

7. The current should be turned on and the dial adjusted to the highest point or the highest reading which can be obtained without streams of bubbles rising to the surface of the electroplating solution from the electrodes.

8. The electroplating unit should be left on for twelve to fifteen hours to produce an even coating of silver, and at the end of this time the current should be turned off and the plated impression removed.

9. A cast may now be prepared in the plated impression. When

the cast is removed from the impression, the metal plate will come off with the cast.

Uses for Police

The electroplating technique will provide an extremely accurate metal-coated cast which is very useful in recording the distinctive ridges left by a tooth as it bites into a perishable object, such as a piece of fruit, cheese, or candy, for comparison under a binocular comparison microscope with a similar bite mark obtained from a suspect into a similar object, several weeks to several months later.

It is very important that plated dies be made of perishable items of physical evidence because due to the very nature of some of these items and due to the length of time between the time this particular piece of evidence is discovered and the time the suspect is apprehended, the original object may have decomposed, changed or degenerated to such a degree that no comparison can be made. If a highly accurate polysulfide rubber impression is taken of the piece of physical evidence in question, and if a highly accurate metalized silver or copper cast is prepared, then there will be something to compare with the suspect's tooth marks into a similar substance.

Although this technique is easy, it is time-consuming and for this reason should be reserved strictly for use with perishable items of physical evidence.

Chapter 8 _ _ _ _ _ _ _ _ _

TRAY MATERIALS AND TECHNIQUES

_ _ _ _ _ _ _ _ _ _ _ _ _

A TRAY is a piece of plastic or metal formed to approximately fit an item of physical evidence, a part of the body, or a dental arch and is used to carry impression material and hold it against said object. A tray may either be *stock*, that is, manufactured in a standard, preformed shape of a dental arch; or it may be *custom*, or individually made to closely fit a particular object. Stock trays are used in most cases when the impression is to be taken in the mouth with certain materials. Custom trays are constructed to fit items of physical evidence or parts of the body outside the mouth, and in certain special instances the dental arch.

In cases when a custom tray is to be constructed for use inside the mouth, a written work order, signed by a licensed dentist must be obtained. Additionally, when the impression is actually taken with any of the trays, the laws and rules described in Chapter 6 should be carefully observed.

STOCK TRAYS

The stock tray is a mass-produced form of metal or plastic, either perforated or unperforated, suitable for holding and carrying impression material to the mouth and manufactured in a number of sizes, graded numerically from the largest down to the smallest. They may be purchased from most dental supply houses in kits containing the various size gradations.

Trays for Impression Plaster

Type and Appearance

Stock trays for plaster are single pieces of unperforated metal shaped to roughly conform to the outline of the teeth and dental

arches. They contain a handle made of the same material, and somewhere on the handle is generally stamped a number indicating the
size of the tray.

Reasons for this Construction

Stock trays for use with impression plaster are made of unperforated sheet metal because when impression plaster is placed in the
mouth it flows into all of the spaces between the teeth and around
the teeth, and when the material sets, it locks itself into place and
must be fractured carefully in order to remove it. If the stock tray
has perforations with bits of plaster sticking through, thus holding
the tray against the plaster material, it will be impossible, or at least
very difficult, to remove the tray from the plaster without completely destroying the impression.

The unperforated stock tray can be removed, leaving the plaster
impression in place in the mouth, after which the impression may be
carefully scored and fractured off the teeth and reassembled in the
tray. The stock tray will contain various lines and ridges roughly
corresponding to the lines of the teeth and the dental arches in general which will make it easy to align the fragments in the tray prior
to pouring the material up with the chosen cast material.

Method of Selection

The selection of a stock tray for use with plaster is very simple.
The smallest size of tray which will go into the mouth and which,
when in place in the mouth, will cover all of the teeth from the back
of the farthest back tooth on one side to the back of the farthest
back tooth on the other side, upper or lower, should be selected. The
flanges, or outside edges of the upper tray and the outside and inside
areas of the lower tray may be bent so the metal is not resting directly against the gums. A space of approximately one-fourth inch
should be allowed between all areas of the impression tray and the
objects in the mouth.

Trays for Nonreversible Hydrocolloid
(Alginate) Impression Material

Types and Appearances

There are a number of types of stock trays intended for use with alginate, most of which fit into the three categories of trays described and evaluated below.

PERFORATED METAL TRAY. The first type of stock tray intended for use with alginate is the perforated metal tray. This is a piece of heavy wire or perforated sheet metal shaped to conform to an outline of the teeth and the supporting dental arches. The rims of the tray are enclosed with a heavy piece of round wire soldered to the heavy metal screen or perforated metal. There is also a handle attached to the front part of the tray made of solid sheet metal. The size of the stock tray is generally stamped somewhere on this handle.

PERFORATED PLASTIC TRAY WITH FEW LARGE HOLES. Another type of tray for use with alginate is the perforated plastic tray with only a few large holes. It is made from a solid sheet of plastic shaped to conform to the dental arch and teeth and into which have been punched approximately four to eight holes of one-fourth inch diameter. On the upper tray the holes are scattered over the area of the biting surfaces of the teeth and across the roof of the mouth, and in the case of the lower tray, they are placed across the biting surfaces of the teeth only.

PERFORATED PLASTIC TRAY WITH MANY SMALL HOLES. The third type of tray for use with alginate is another type of perforated plastic tray. This tray is made from a solid sheet of plastic perforated by hundreds of tiny holes, perhaps one to one and one-half mm in diameter and scattered all about all surfaces and areas of the impression tray with the exception of the handle.

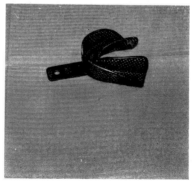

Figure 60. Metal stock tray for use with alginate impression material.

Reasons for this Construction

PERFORATED METAL TRAY. The wire screen or the sheet metal of the perforated metal tray has thousands of perforations which allow the alginate material to squeeze through and diffuse together joining the impression tray tightly and firmly to the mass of the impression itself, so that when the impression tray is removed from the mouth the mass of the impression is removed with it.

Metal trays are durable and may be cleaned, sterilized and reused with little deterioration. The only disadvantage of the stock metal tray is that after the tray is used for some time, the appearance of the tray becomes marred by tarnish.

PERFORATED PLASTIC TRAY WITH FEW LARGE HOLES. The idea behind perforated plastic trays containing only a small number of relatively large holes is that the small number of large holes will allow enough alginate to be expressed through to hold the tray against the alginate so the tray may be removed from the mouth containing the alginate impression; by having a relatively few number of holes, the tray is supposed to hold and force larger amounts of the alginate impression material into more of the nooks and crannies in the mouth, producing a more accurate impression.

The perforated plastic tray containing few holes has a significant disadvantage. In most instances, with most alginate hydrocolloid materials, the small number of large holes is inadequate to hold the stock

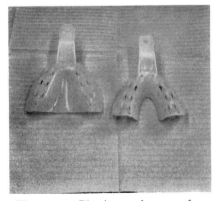

Figure 61. Plastic stock trays for use with alginate impression material.

tray against the impression material, and often when this type of stock tray is removed from the mouth, the impression will stay in contact with the teeth. When this happens the alginate impression must be carefully removed from the teeth, and the risk of fracturing the impression or distorting it beyond repair is great. The perforated plastic tray with a few large holes, if used, must be coated with an adhesive prior to loading it with alginate impression material. The use of this type of stock tray is not recommended.

PERFORATED PLASTIC TRAY WITH MANY SMALL HOLES. The intention of constructing a perforated plastic tray with a large number of small holes is to allow the alginate impression material to be squeezed through the thousands of tiny holes and to join together into a mass which tightly holds the impression tray against the impression so that the impression may be removed from the mouth along with the tray easily and with a minimum of distortion.

The disadvantage of the perforated plastic tray containing a large number of holes is that in the case of an unusually sized mouth, where it is possible to bend the flanges of a perforated metal tray to accommodate this mouth, it is not possible to bend the flanges of the perforated plastic tray. Occasionally mouths will be either too large or too small to be used with this type of tray.

Method of Selection

A tray should be selected which covers all of the teeth and supporting structures from the back of the farthest rear tooth on one side to the back of the farthest rear tooth on the other side. The impression tray should not rest tightly against the gums but should be away from the gums in all areas for a space of approximately one-fourth inch.

Trays for Polysulfide Rubber Base and Silicone Rubber Base Impression Materials

Type and Appearance

Polysulfide rubber base and silicone rubber base impression materials are used with identical types of trays. A stock tray intended for use with these impression materials is generally manufactured from a sheet of unperforated plastic shaped to conform to the outline of the teeth and the supporting dental arches. A handle is attached to the front area of the tray and is made of the same material as the tray itself. Somewhere on the handle is usually stamped a number indicating the size of the tray.

Reasons for this Construction

The unperforated plastic stock tray is intended to hold the rubber base impression material and to confine it adequately in place against the structures of the mouth until the material sets. This type of tray is intended to make it unnecessary to construct a custom tray for use with the rubber materials.

Rubber and silicone base impression materials are more sensitive to the amount of thickness left for the material between the tooth and the tray than are most other impression materials, the best range being a distance of about one-fourth inch. If more space is allowed, the rubber impression material may not adequately support the weight of the cast material with which the impression is poured, and there may be a resultant sagging and distortion. Most stock trays intended for use with rubber base or silicone impression materials allow for a much greater distance than one-fourth inch between the tooth and the seat of the tray, allowing for this distortion to occur. For this reason stock trays are not recommended for use with rubber base or silicone impression materials.

Method of Selection

If it is necessary for some unusual reason to use a stock tray with rubber base or silicone rubber base impression materials, a tray should be selected which extends from the farthest back area of the farthest rear tooth on the one side to the farthest back area of the farthest rear tooth on the other side. All teeth and all other areas of the arch should be covered. The tray should allow for a one-fourth inch space between the teeth and other areas of the supporting arches and the material composing the tray itself.

Uses for Police

Stock trays generally may be used with impression plaster, nonreversible hydrocolloid (alginate) impression material, and in very rare instances, with rubber base or silicone rubber base impression materials, for purposes of taking impressions in the mouth when a record of moderate accuracy is desired, including those instances when the dentist will analyze and compare the casts with other casts and other records. They may also be used to take impressions of the dental arches at autopsy for record purposes and as an aid in determining dental identification of unclaimed bodies.

CUSTOM TRAYS

A custom tray is an individually constructed tray of solid plastic, sheet metal, perforated metal or wire, or cold-cure acrylic constructed outside the mouth and contoured to closely fit the dental arch or any object outside of the mouth or any part of the body of which an accurate impression is desired. A custom tray may be easily and quickly prepared by the officer or technician at the scene or elsewhere. The tray should carry the proper amount of impression material to the object; that is, it should allow for an even amount of space so that the thickness of impression material is uniform throughout, not exceeding one-fourth inch. It should be contoured to fit the shape of the object of the impression to result in a thinner and more uniform layer of impression material and minimize distortion. This is important because some materials, particularly silicone impression material, shrink to a varying degree over a period of hours. As this shrinkage varies according to the thickness of the material, if the material is not of uniform thickness, the shrinkage will be greater in some areas of the impression than others and distortions will result.

Custom Trays for Impression Plaster

Type and Appearance

A custom tray for impression plaster consists of a piece of medium gauge sheet metal which is cut with tin snips and bent and fashioned with contouring pliers to the outline of the object of the impression. The border of this type of tray is crimped inwards toward the center, approximately one-fourth to one-half inch at one-inch intervals around the edges of the tray. This type of tray is used for impressions of portions of the body outside the mouth.

Reasons for this Construction

A custom tray intended for use with plaster impression material must not contain any perforations to hold the tray to the plaster in order to allow the tray to be removed separately from the plaster impression, carefully scored and fractured, and reassembled in the tray. The crimpings around the edge are to aid in the reassembly of the plaster impression in the tray after it has been fractured away from the object of the impression.

Techniques of Construction

To construct a custom tray for use with plaster, the following materials are needed:

1. a sheet of medium gauge, unperforated metal, which is workable enough to be bent with pliers and cut with tin snips;
2. a pair of heavy tin snips; and
3. a pair of heavy round, or half-round electrical pliers with which to contour the sheet metal and crimp the borders.

The tray is constructed in the following manner:

1. The sheet metal should be held above the object of which the impression will be taken. With the tin snips the metal should be cut so that the sheet metal covers an area perhaps one-third larger than the area to be included in the impression.
2. With the round or half-round heavy electrical pliers, the sheet metal should be carefully shaped and contoured so that it roughly follows the outline and contour of the object.
3. The edge of the border of the tray should be grasped with ap-

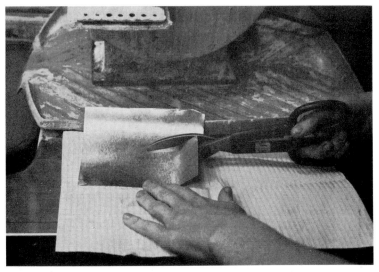

Figure 62. Cutting sheet metal to the proper size for a custom tray for use with impression plaster.

proximately one-fourth to one-half inch of the tip of the pliers and the pliers should be moved sharply inwards at intervals ranging from one-fourth to one inch, making an edge approxi-

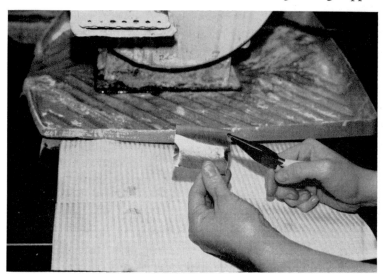

Figure 63. The edges of the plaster tray are crimped after the tray has been roughly formed to the shape of the object of which the impression is to be made.

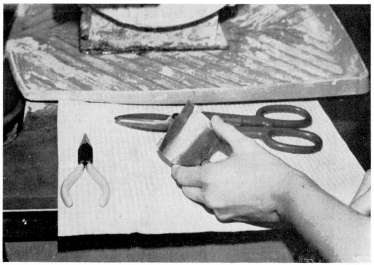

Figure 64. A completed custom tray for use with impression plaster.

mately perpendicular to the tray, depending on the size of the object of the impression. This will aid in the reassembly of the fractured plaster back inside the tray after it has been removed from the object.

4. The impression plaster may now be loaded into the custom tray.

Custom Trays for Nonreversible Hydrocolloid (Alginate) Impression Material

Type and Appearance

Custom trays intended for use with alginate impression material are made from medium to heavy gauge wire screen of a type which can be cut with heavy tin snips. The medium-to-heavy gauge screen is contoured roughly to the shape and form of the object of the impression. The edges of the tray are aligned with a thin rope (one-fourth inch diameter) of cold-cure acrylic and a handle, also of cold-cure acrylic, may be fastened somewhere in the center of the tray or at one of the edges. This type of tray is generally used for impressions of portions of the body outside the mouth or objects of physical evidence.

Reasons for this Construction

Medium-to-heavy gauge wire screening is used to provide a number of holes and perforations through which the alginate material can be expressed and can go together holding the impression tray firmly against the alginate when the impression sets so the tray can be removed with the impression in one piece. The rope of cold-cure acrylic around the edge of the tray is intended to reinforce the tray and hold it in position after it has been shaped to conform to the outlines of the object of the impression. The acrylic handle is intended to aid in the removal of the tray with the impression.

Techniques of Construction

To construct a custom tray for alginate impression material the following materials are necessary:

1. a large piece of medium-to-heavy gauge wire screening;
2. a pair of heavy tin snips;
3. a pair of heavy, round-beaked or half-round-beaked electrical pliers;

4. a small porcelain or glass container with a lid; this will be used to contain the mixture of acrylic for the rim;

5. a small mixing spatula with rounded ends and a flat blade, the blade being no more than one-fourth inch wide at its widest point, and not flexible;

6. an eyedropper;

7. a measuring device to measure the proper amount of the polymer and the monomer of acrylic; and

8. bottles of acrylic monomer and polymer ingredients.

The following are the steps in the construction of a custom tray for use with alginate:

1. A piece of the wire screen, approximately one-third larger than

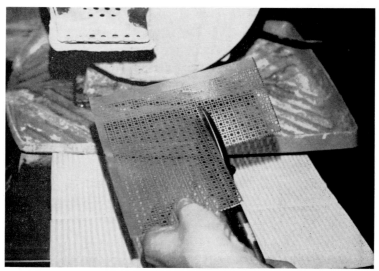

Figure 65. Perforated sheet metal being cut for a custom tray for use with alginate impression material.

the area of the impression, should be cut with the tin snips.

2. Using the round-beaked or half-round-beaked electrical pliers, the wire screen should be shaped and formed to conform to the outlines of the object of the impression. The screen should be placed on any convenient surface except the object or person of which the impression is to be made.

3. Cold-cure acrylic should be prepared as described in the section on acrylics in Chapter 7 in an amount adequate to provide

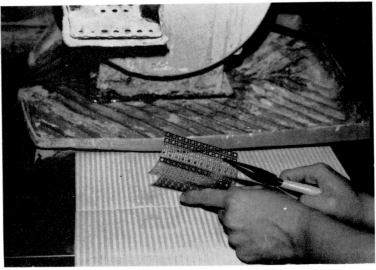

Figure 66. Contouring of a custom tray for use with alginate.

a border for the screen and a handle. The precautions advised regarding this material should be carefully observed.

4. When the acrylic is of a putty-like consistency, it should be removed from the mixing jar and on the large pad of linoleum

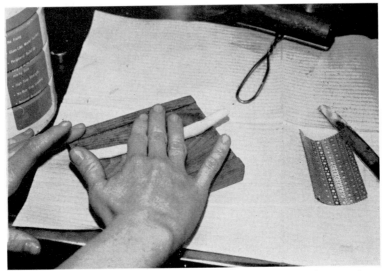

Figure 67. Acrylic rope being prepared to form a reinforcing border and handle for an alginate custom tray.

or heavy oiled paper, rolled into a long rope. This rope should be placed on the edge of the contoured wire screening and gently pressed into the wire screen. The screen should not be filled in; only the edge should be reinforced.

5. If acrylic is left over, as some should be, it should be rolled into a thick ball or mass and pressed with the fingers so that it is in a

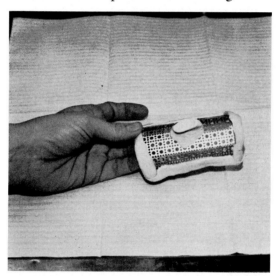

Figure 68. Finished alginate custom tray, top view.

more or less cylindrical shape, and this should be pressed through the wire screen of the custom tray so that bits of the acrylic are forced onto the other side. The other side should be patted so that the acrylic is flattened out against the screen on the other side. This piece of acrylic will serve as a handle.

6. The acrylic should be allowed to set.

7. The custom tray is ready for use with an alginate hydrocolloid impression material.

Custom Trays for Polysulfide Rubber Base or Silicone Rubber Base Impression Materials

Types and Appearances

A custom tray intended for use with polysulfide rubber base impression or silicone rubber base impression material is made from a

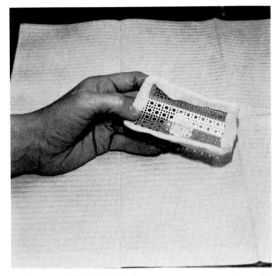

Figure 69. Finished alginate custom tray, viewed from the reverse side.

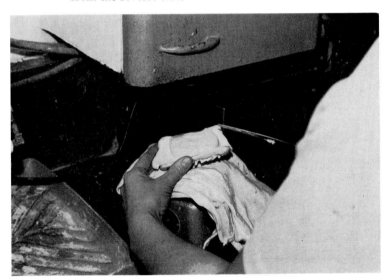

Figure 70. Pouring stone into an alginate impression made with a custom tray.

thin piece of plastic, usually cold-cure acrylic, which is closely fitted to the object of which the impression is to be taken. It is unperforated and contains a handle made of the same type of acrylic as the rest of the tray attached in a noncritical area. If the object of the impression is relatively large, there are two or three small extensions on the side of the tray towards the object the impression will be taken of, which will rest in noncritical areas on the object to insure a one-quarter-inch thickness of the impression material. A custom tray rather than a stock tray is almost always used with rubber or silicone rubber base impression material.

Reasons for this Construction

A custom tray intended for use with rubber base or silicone base impression materials is not perforated because once this type of impression material sets it is very difficult, if not impossible, to remove it from a perforated tray because the impression sets into a solid mass of rubber. The material would have to be cut away slowly and meticulously with a razor blade, scalpel blade, or similar instrument and would take a great deal of time. Consequently, this type of custom tray is painted with an adhesive included by the manufacturer in the rubber base or silicone base impression material kit to make the impression material adhere to the tray.

Since the reason for taking a polysulfide rubber impression or a silicone rubber impression is the accuracy, custom trays are usually made in lieu of using stock trays, both outside and inside the mouth, to assure the uniform thickness of the material necessary to prevent distortions.

Cold-cure acrylics are used instead of unperforated sheet metal for the construction of custom trays intended for use with polysulfide rubber base or silicone rubber base impression materials because both polysulfide rubber base and silicone rubber base impression materials are very tough, strong, and resilient materials which set up in contact with an object. When these materials are pulled away from the object against which they are lying, a partial vacuum is created, and as the material is pulled harder, the stresses within the material tend to pull the tray back toward the object. The forces generated are often great enough to bend a metal tray, but the cold-cure acrylic will stand stresses of this magnitude without appreciable distortion.

Techniques of Construction

The following materials are needed to construct a custom tray for use with rubber base or silicone base impression materials:

1. a small porcelain or glass container with a lid, to mix acrylic for the tray;
2. a small spatula with rounded ends and a flat inflexible blade, no more than one-fourth inch wide at its widest point;
3. an eyedropper;
4. a measuring device to measure the proper amount of the polymer and the monomer of acrylic;
5. bottles of acrylic monomer and acrylic polymer ingredients;
6. a small camelhair brush;
7. a large (6" x 6") slick linoleum tile or glass slab or pad of heavy oiled paper;
8. several sheets or strips of asbestos or several sheets or strips of pink base plate wax.
9. If the custom tray to be fabricated is intended for use in the mouth, plaster models (casts) of the subject's upper and lower teeth are needed. These should be made from alginate impressions taken with stock trays in the standard manner.

The following are the steps in the construction of a custom tray for use with polysulfide rubber base impression material or silicone base impression material:

FOR USE ON AN OBJECT OR PART OF THE BODY OUTSIDE OF THE MOUTH:

1. A layer approximately one-fourth inch thick of either asbestos or pink base plate wax should be placed over the area the impression is to be taken of.
2. Using the blunt end of the spatula, two or more holes should be scraped in noncritical areas of the impression (not over the bite mark or tooth indentation) so that small extensions of acrylic from the tray will actually contact the object of the impression to insure that the tray gets no closer than one-fourth inch away from the surface of the object, thus assuring an ideal thickness of the rubber base material.
3. Cold-cure acrylic in an amount large enough to cover the prospective tray area should be prepared in the manner described in the acrylic section of Chapter 7. Attention should be paid to the precautions regarding the use of this material.
4. When the cold-cure acrylic has reached a putty-like consistency, the acrylic should be removed from the mixing jar and

placed on a pad of linoleum or heavy oiled paper and set aside for one minute.

5. The acrylic that is on the linoleum pad or the pad of heavy oiled paper or the glass slab should be gently rolled into a cylinder one-half inch longer than the length or width of the object the custom tray is being made for.

6. Enough acrylic from one end or another of this cylinder should be cut off with the spatula to make the cylinder conform roughly to the length or width of the object of the custom tray. The extra piece should be set aside; it will be used later to make the handle.

7. The cylinder should be placed upon the object of the impression, and with gentle but firm finger pressure the putty-like acrylic should be molded over the entire area covered by the asbestos or wax with care to not extend over the area covered by the asbestos or wax. Enough pressure should be used to force a small amount of the acrylic plastic through the small holes scraped in the asbestos or the wax to provide stops to insure the ideal amount of space between the surface of the tray and the surface of the object.

8. The small camelhair brush should be dipped into the cold-cure monomer and a thin layer of the monomer should be painted on an area of the tray which appears to be a convenient place to attach a handle; with the camelhair brush, a small amount of the cold-cure monomer should be painted over the small tag of acrylic which was cut off the end of the cylinder before the cylinder of acrylic was used to make the tray. This small remnant of acrylic should be attached to the tray so that the areas of the acrylic remnant and the tray which were both painted with the monomer are in contact. This will cause the two pieces of acrylic to permanently fuse when they have set, so the handle will not come off when the tray is removed.

9. When the tray material begins to feel very hot and firm it should quickly but gently be removed from the object for which the tray is being made and set aside.

10. After the tray has cooled, indicating that the setting reaction has ended, the layer of asbestos or wax should be scraped off the inside of the custom tray with the end of the spatula, the

side of a blade of a pocket knife or any similar type of scraper.

11. The adhesive supplied with the impression material should be coated in a thin layer onto the entire inside of the tray (the part of the tray which will be facing the surface of the object). The tray is now ready for use.

FOR USE IN THE MOUTH:

1. The upper and lower casts of the subject's upper and lower teeth should be covered with enough sheets of asbestos or pink base plate wax to provide a layer one-fourth inch thick. The asbestos or wax should cover all of the teeth.

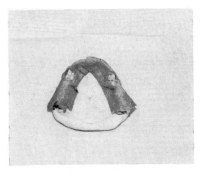

Figure 71. A preliminary cast, covered with asbestos with two stops scraped out over the premolar areas.

2. Using the end of the spatula, two small holes should be scraped through the noncritical areas (which are most likely to be at the back since most bite marks are left by the front teeth). One hole on either side (right and left) should be scraped through the asbestos or the base plate wax so that when the acrylic material is placed over this, pieces of acrylic will be forced through into contact with the teeth to insure that the surface of the tray will be at least one-fourth inch away from the surface of the teeth.

3. Cold-cure acrylic in an amount large enough to cover the prospective tray area should be prepared in the manner described in the acrylic section of Chapter 7. Attention should be paid to the precautions regarding the use of this material.

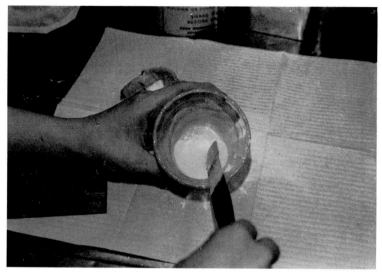

Figure 72. A very large batch of cold cure acrylic being mixed.

4. When the cold-cure acrylic has reached a putty-like consistency, the acrylic should be removed from the mixing jar and placed on a pad of linoleum or heavy oiled paper and set aside for one minute.

5. The putty-like acrylic should be rolled into a rope long enough to reach from the back of the farthest back tooth on one side of the arch to the back of the farthest back tooth on the other side of the arch. Then the roll should be lengthened until it is approximately one-half inch longer.

6. The extra amount of acrylic should be cut off and set aside; it will be used to construct the handle.

7. The rope of acrylic should be placed over the top of the biting surfaces of all of the teeth, from the farthest back tooth on one side to the farthest back tooth on the other side. If there are teeth missing, the rope of acrylic should go from the farthest back tooth on one side to a point on the other side of the cast directly opposite that tooth.

8. Using gentle finger pressure, this rope of plastic should be molded until it covers all areas covered by the asbestos or pink wax. Gently but firmly the plastic should be molded until the surface is reasonably smooth and the pieces of plastic

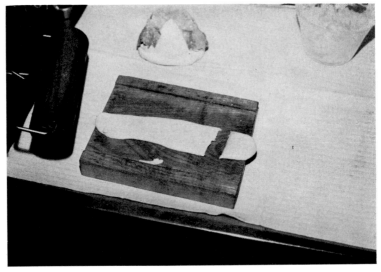

Figure 73. A formed rope of cold cure acrylic in the dough stage, flattened and ready for use. The small part to the right is used to form a handle.

are forced through the holes in the asbestos or pink wax placed there by the blade of the spatula to provide stops to keep the surface of the tray one-fourth inch away from the surface of the teeth.

9. With the small camelhair brush, a small coat of monomer liquid should be painted over an area of approximately one inch on the front of the tray and on a portion of the small remnant piece of acrylic that was cut off the rope before it was placed on the teeth of the cast. The remnant piece should be placed over the area of the tray painted with the cold-cure monomer so that the two areas painted with monomer are in contact and pressed firmly together. This will form the handle.

10. The acrylic will begin to get very hot. When the acrylic no longer feels very hot to the touch, it may be removed from the cast.

11. Using the end of the spatula, the edge of a pocket knife blade or any similar type of scraper, all remnants of the asbestos sheet or the pink base wax should be carefully removed from the inside of the impression tray.

12. The entire inside of the tray should be painted with a thin layer of the adhesive included with the impression material. The custom tray is now ready for use in the mouth.

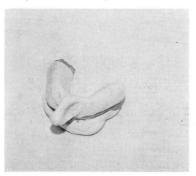

Figure 74. A finished acrylic custom tray for use with silicone or polysulfide rubber base impression material.

Uses for Police

Custom trays are required in the following situations:

1. When an extremely accurate rubber base or silicone base impression is needed for an extremely accurate cast of the human dental arches for purposes of comparison by the dentist;
2. When an impression is desired of any bite marks, indentations, raised welts, or any other tooth-inflicted injuries found on any portion of the human body.
3. When an impression is desired of a piece of perishable physical evidence so that a permanent record of the bite mark may be obtained.
4. For situations when a bite mark is made into a relatively firm material, such as cheese or certain types of candy, leaving striations from the edges of the teeth, so that plated impressions can be made for binocular comparison microscope comparisons with bite marks made in a similar type of material by a suspect at a later date;
5. To obtain impressions for the construction of the cast for record purposes or for analysis or comparison from autopsy material;
6. On any occasions when the dentist requests that a custom tray be used.

Appendix I
BINOCULAR COMPARISON MICROSCOPE

The binocular comparison microscope is very rarely used in the field of dental evidence, and its use is limited to only one type of case. For that reason, the information relating to this piece of equipment has been placed in the Appendix. It is, however, very valuable in the rare instances its use may be called upon, and no text on dental evidence would be complete without mention of it.

The binocular comparison microscope is basically two separate microscopes mounted beside each other and attached by a comparison bridge on which there are a series of lenses which fuse the images produced by objects as they appear beneath the scope of each of the microscopes. Under each scope, there is a small holder which can be rotated, causing the object being examined to be rotated.

This type of microscope is useful in ballistics for examination of bullet slugs for striations, for comparison of marks made by tools, and for comparison examinations of miscellaneous types of trace evidence with control samples of similar materials in an effort to place an individual at the scene of the crime by virtue of the presence at the scene of the crime of these items of trace evidence.

In dental forensics, the binocular comparison microscope is used to compare the marks made by the incision teeth into firm or semi firm objects such as cheese or various types of candy or other items of physical evidence which may have been bitten by the suspect, with similar items of similar consistency which have been deliberately bitten by the suspect under experimental conditions after his apprehension. An attempt is made to find the similarities of scratches left by the teeth in or on the objects viewed under the microscope. The items of physical evidence, or as is more often the case the items of experimental evidence and the electroplated models of the items of physical evidence, are rotated until a relative match is found

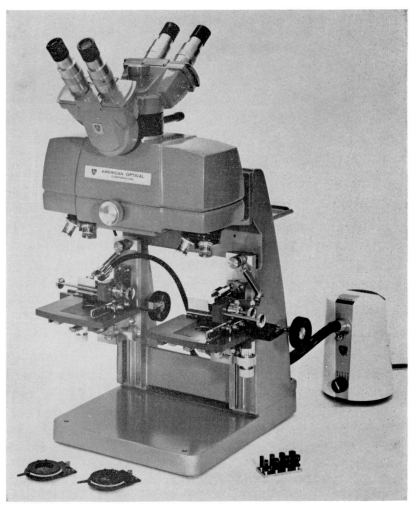

Figure 75. Binocular comparison microscope. (Courtesy of American Optical Corporation, Scientific Instruments Division, Buffalo, New York.)

between the stripes or scratches on one object and the stripes or scratches on the other.

A picture then is taken through the lens of the microscope, and this picture, referred to as a photomicrograph, is obtained.

TYPES OF CASES

The binocular comparison microscope is used exclusively in cases where bite marks have been left in items of physical evidence which are solid and firm enough to allow a clear imprint of the scratches made by the teeth as they bite into or through the item.

Teeth, since they are used in biting and tearing, are subjected to stresses and strains in excess of 500 pounds per square inch, and they become worn and nicked unevenly at their biting edges. These nicks in turn leave distinctive marks when they are used to bite into a reasonably firm material. The nicks or scratches or striations may be of great importance in determining whether or not the incision was made by a specific individual, especially in cases where the results of tests have proved inconclusive. The objects of physical evidence bearing these tooth marks or striations are generally articles of food left at the scene of the crime. The materials which will hold this type of striation are generally cheeses of the firm or semifirm variety, pieces of candy, and pieces of chewing gum. Pieces of chewing gum are notoriously unreliable because of the distortion of the scratches or striations caused by the elasticity of the chewing gum itself, although occasionally there is a good piece. The examination of chewing gum under the comparison microscope will in most cases prove inconclusive.

Procedures

Although the dentist should examine any and all photomicrographs made of the physical evidence and the sample, the actual operation and examination of the material under the binocular comparison microscope may be carried out by an evidence technician, any specifically trained police officer, or the dentist himself. The exact techniques involved in the use of the instrument have not been included, as they may be found in any text of evidence technology. The instances when the dentist will use the binocular comparison microscope will be few and far between because most dentists are not trained in the operation of this piece of equipment. If the dentist wishes to examine the objects of evidence under the binocular comparison microscope and has had little or no experience with this piece of equipment, the principles of operation closely enough resemble those examinations under more conventional microscopes with which he is familiar, so that with a minimum of coaching from the evidence technician, the dentist will be able to adequately use this device.

Following are procedures for the police technician to follow in using this microscope in dental evidence cases:

1. When an item of physical evidence bearing tooth imprints or scratches is found, and a suspect is apprehended, it will be necessary to obtain either the suspect's informed consent or a court order for the following procedure.

2. The suspect should be asked to bite into an object as similar as possible to that found at the scene of the crime, or in lieu of that, into a large piece of firm pink wax.

3. The severed end of the physical evidence which has been bitten should be placed under one end of the binocular comparison microscope, and the incised area of the recently bitten sample placed under the other barrel. If the object of physical evidence with which the comparison is to be made is perishable, as is generally the case, an electroplated cast of an impression of the physical evidence may be substituted for the original.

4. The entire surface either of the cast of the physical evidence or the original physical evidence should be examined in detail at low magnification to locate the most prominent group of markings; when found this item is allowed to become stationary.

5. The recently obtained test sample, whether it is of wax or of a material similar to that originally bitten, should then be manipulated in an attempt to find a similar area with the same characteristics which match those on the evidence material.

6. If and when a match is found, both the sample of evidence and the recently obtained test sample should be manipulated in an attempt to find out whether or not similar coincidental marks are found in other areas of the two items.

7. If similar marks are found while the test sample and the sample of evidence or the cast of evidence are in the same relative position as when the first coordinates were made, all markings on both samples should be examined at a higher magnification.

8. A careful and detailed study of all the details on both samples will eventually permit the technician to conclude that the incision marks were either made or not made by the same person.

9. When the technician finds areas that match more closely than any others, a picture can be taken by a camera attached to the

microscope, the photomicrograph, to show and record this comparison. Many comparative micrography experts do not use these photomicrographs as demonstrative evidence in court, however. Instead, the test procedures they have followed are explained in detail along with the conclusions they have reached, without the use of any illustrative exhibits, because occasionally the evidence with the incision marks or striations may be so distorted and twisted that not all of them may be in focus in the photomicrograph, resulting in blurred areas, or to a layman, apparent discrepancies even when these discrepancies do not in fact exist.

Uses for Police

The binocular comparison microscope is useful in the examination of pieces of physical trace evidence consisting of candy, cheese or other firm objects left at the scene of the crime in comparison with similar objects bitten experimentally at a later date by the suspect. The results of this type of examination will not be in the nature of incriminating evidence, but rather in the nature of supporting evidence which will not in itself be sufficient to convict, but can place the suspect definitely at the scene of the crime. The information obtained from this type of examination can also be used as a lever in the process of interrogation in an attempt to obtain a confession from the suspect.

Appendix II
AVERAGE DATES OF TOOTH ERUPTION

6 Months
lower central incisor

7 Months
upper central incisor
lower lateral incisor

8 Months
upper lateral incisor

1 Year
lower first primary molar

1½ Years
lower cuspid
upper cuspid
upper first primary molar

2 Years
lower second primary molar
upper second primary molar

6 Years
lower central incisor
lower first permanent molar
upper first permanent molar

7 Years
upper central incisor
lower lateral incisor

8 Years
upper lateral incisor

10 Years
lower first premolar
upper first premolar
lower cuspid

12 Years
lower second premolar
upper second premolar
upper cuspid
lower second permanent molar
upper second permanent molar

18 to 21 Years
lower third permanent molar
upper third permanent molar

These figures are averages and may vary by as much as nine months either way from the dates indicated. Other information, such as the amount of enamel formed on the unerupted teeth, the degree of root formation, and the degree of closure of the end of the root where the nerve enters the tooth, can give the dentist more clues to determine age from the teeth.

Appendix III
FIELD DENTAL EVIDENCE KIT

Graphite pencil
Red and blue pencil
Ink eraser
1 bottle of green soap
Dental mirrors
3 straight probes
3 curved probes
3 clear plastic bags (large)
3 clear plastic bags (small)
1 glass mixing slab
Pack of department's dental charts
3 pair cotton pliers
3 labeled specimen bottles with
    10% formalin
3 labeled, stoppered test tubes
1 box of large cotton pellets
1 jar of distilled water
1 box of absorbent paper sheets
Camera Equipment:
    35 mm camera loaded with
        black-and-white-film
    35 mm camera loaded with color
        film
    35 mm camera loaded with
        infrared film
    red and blue filters
    a flash attachment

3 sizes, upper stock alginate trays
3 sizes, lower stock alginate trays
1′ x 1′ unperforated sheet metal
1′ x 1′ heavy wire screen
1 roll, asbestos strips
1 rubber mixing bowl
1 flexible alginate spatula
5 packets of alginate impression
    material with powder and
    liquid measures
1 Polysulfide rubber base impres-
    sion material kit, regular type
1 pair tin snips
1 pair straight-nose electrical pliers
1 millimeter ruler, 5 cm long
1 acrylic kit, with powder and
    liquid measures and mixing jar

Appendix IV

STATES IN WHICH DESIGNATED ASSISTANTS MAY TAKE IMPRESSIONS FOR RECORDS

The states listed below allow dental assistants to legally take impressions for record purposes. In some this is due to provisions in the Dental Practice Act. In others it is allowed under administrative regulations made by the State Dental Board, but which are not part of the practice act. This list is growing yearly, so check your own state's current regulations to be sure. Some States' Boards not listed here may allow police to take impressions for forensic purposes in instances when there is a clear need for casts as evidence, especially if this is requested by a state's attorney for the police department. This, however, should never be assumed, and the Dental Board in question should be approached first before the need arises. In all other states all impressions in the mouth must be made by a licensed dentist, although anyone may take impressions of parts of the body or objects outside the mouth and prepare casts from impressions when a signed work order is given by a licensed dentist.

Alabama	R	Missouri	R	U. S. Armed Forces	
Alaska	A	New Mexico	R	U. S. Public Health	
Colorado	A	Oklahoma	R	Service	
Delaware	R	Pennsylvania	R	U. S. Coast &	
Florida	R	South Dakota	R	Geodetic Survey	
Iowa	R	Tennessee	A	bases and vessels.	
Kansas	A	Washington	A		
Kentucky	R	Wisconsin	R		
Minnesota	R	Wyoming	R		
Mississippi	A	Puerto Rico	R		

R=Allowed under Rules and Regulations of the State Dental Board
A=Allowed specifically in the State Dental Practice Act

BIBLIOGRAPHY

CHAPTER 1

Noble, L.: Notes on the trial of Professor Webster for the murder of Dr. Parkman. *J Baltimore Coll Dent Surg*, May, 1962.

CHAPTER 2

Guyton, A.C.: *Medical Physiology*. Philadelphia, Saunders, 1964.

Keiser-Nielsen, S.: Geographic factors in forensic odontology. *Int Dent J*, 15:343-347, 1965.

Lasker, G.W., and Lee, M.C.: Racial traits in the human teeth. *J Forens Sci*, 2:401-419, 1957.

Ramfjord, S., and Ash, M.M.: *Occlusion*. Philadelphia, Saunders, 1966.

Sicher, Harry: *Oral Anatomy*, 3rd ed. St. Louis, Mosby, 1960.

Wheeler, R.: *A Textbook of Dental Anatomy and Physiology*, 5th ed. Philadelphia, Saunders, 1974.

Woodburne, R.T.: *Essentials of Human Anatomy*. New York, Oxford, 1961.

CHAPTER 3

Butler, O.H.: The value of bite mark evidence. *International Journal of Forensic Odontology*, Vol. 1, No. 2, Oct., 1973.

Camps, F.E.: *Medical and Scientific Investigations in the Christie Case*. London, Medical Publications, 1953.

Danielson, Knud: The battered child syndrome. *Newsletter of the Scandinavian Society of Forensic Odontology*, 6:93-98, 1972.

Furahata, T., and Yamamoto, K.: *Forensic Odontology*. Springfield, Thomas, 1967.

Glaister, J., and Brash, J.C.: *Medico-Legal Aspects of the Ruxton Case* (The Dental Evidence of Investigation). Edinburgh, Livingstone, 1937, pp. 1-19, 84-88, 102-103, 121-126.

Gustafson, Gösta: *Forensic Odontology*. New York, Elsevier, 1966.

Keiser–Nielsen, S.: Dental identification in mass disasters. *J Dent Res, 42*: 303-311, 1963.

Keiser–Nielsen, S., Frykholm, K.O., and Ström, F.: Identification of unknown bodies: Procedures used in Scandinavia, emphasizing odontological aspects. *Int Dent J, 14*:317-329, 1964.

Keyes, F.: Teeth marks in the skin as evidence in establishing identity. *Dental Cosmos, 67*:1165-1167, 1925.

Levine, L.J.: The solution of a battered child homicide by dental evidence. *J Am Dent Assoc*, Vol. 86, No. 61, 1973, pp. 1234-1237.

186

Luntz, Lester, and Luntz, Phyllis: *Handbook of Dental Identification.* Philadelphia, Lippincott, 1973.

Nickolls, L.C.: Identification by tooth marks. *The Police Journal*, 23:263-264, 1950.

Powell, T.G.E.: *Barclodiad y Gawres.* Liverpool, Liverpool Press, pp. 62-69, 1956.

Simpson, K.: Dental evidence in the reconstruction of crime. *Br Dent J*, 91: 229-238, 1951.

————: Dental data in crime investigation. *Criminal Police Review*, 6:312-317, 1951.

Voorhies, J.: Crime detection through dentistry: Identification of Grace Budd made by two New York dentists. *Oral Hygiene*, 25:1085-1093, 1935.

CHAPTER 4

Adlington, J.A., and Rosen, J.G.: Identification by dental records. *Supple ment Army Medical Bulletin, The Dental Bulletin*, 11:103, 1940.

Frykholm, K.O., and Lysell, L.: Different systems for the recording of teeth and teeth surfaces. *Int Dent J*, 12:194-207, 1962.

Humble, B.H.: Identification by means of the teeth. *Br Dent J*, 54:528-536, 1933.

Lyon, H.W.: Use of intraoral photographs as a means of personnel identification and registration of oral lesions and deformities. *Research Report, Project NM-008-012. 03. 04*, 11:693-741, Naval Medical Center, Bethesda, 1953.

————: An intraoral photographic apparatus for personnel identification. *U. S. Forces Medical Journal*, 10:304-311, 1959.

Montagu, Ashley: *A Handbook of Anthropometry.* Springfield, Thomas, 1960.

CHAPTER 5

Arthur, R.: *The Scientific Investigator.* Springfield, Thomas, 1973.

Cornwell, W.S.: Radiographic and photography in problems of identification: A review. *Med Radiogr Photogr*, 32:2, 1956.

Dyce, J.: *Photographic Aids to Clinical Practice.* London, Staples, 1948.

Graham, D., and Grey, H.: The application of X-ray techniques in forensic investigation. *X-Ray Focus*, 6:8-12, 1965.

James, R.A.: Identification of dental X-ray films. *Med Tech Bull*, 6:5-7, 1955.

Morgan, W.D., and Harris, M.C.: The use of X-rays as an aid to medico-legal identification. *J Forensic Med*, 1:28-38, 1953.

O'Brien, R.C., and Frecke, C.L.: Dental Radiography and Dental Photography. *Dental Clinics of North America*, Philadelphia, Saunders, 1968.

O'Hara, C.: *Modern Criminal Investigation.* New York, Funk and Wagnalls, 1962.

CHAPTERS 6, 7, 8

Greener, E.H., Harcourt, J.K., and Lautenschlager, E.P.: *Materials Science in Dentistry.* Baltimore, Wilkins, 1972.

Skinner, E.W., and Phillips, R.W.: *The Science of Dental Materials*, 5th ed. Philadelphia, Saunders, 1960.

INDEX

189